WITHDRAWN

Social Inclusion and Recovery

About the authors

Julie Repper first worked in the mental health service as a nurse. After leaving clinical practice she worked as a lecturer in nursing studies and as a researcher and is now employed as a Senior Research Fellow at the University of Sheffield and as Lead Research Nurse with Community Health Sheffield NHS Trust. In addition to a range of research and service development work, she has a particular interest in promoting user-led research initiatives.

In addition, Julie is a Trustee of Nottingham Advocacy Group and a member of the Board of Governors at the school which her daughters attend, and in this capacity has initiated a 'mental health and emotional well-being' campaign at the school.

Rachel Perkins was a clinical psychologist working in a South London rehabilitation service. After 20 years working within rehabilitation services, as both clinician and Clinical Director, Rachel is now the Clinical Director of Adult Mental Health Services at South West London and St. George's Mental Health NHS Trust and a specialist advisor with the Health Advisory Service. She has a particular interest in disability rights and employment and mental health and established the 'Pathfinder User Employment Programme' – an initiative designed to increase access within mental health services for people who have themselves experienced mental health problems.

As well as her 'day job', Rachel is a member of the Council of the Manic Depression Fellowship and Mental Health Media, and a Member of the Mental Health Action Group of the Disability Rights Commission.

For Churchill Livingstone:

Senior Commissioning Editor: Susan Young
Project Development Manager: Mairi McCubbin
Project Manager: Ailsa Laing
Designer: Judith Wright

Social Inclusion and Recovery

A Model for Mental Health Practice

Julie Repper BA MPhil PhD RMN RGN

Senior Research Fellow, University of Sheffield & Lead Research Nurse, Community Health Sheffield NHS Trust, UK

Rachel Perkins BA MPhil PhD

Clinical Director of General Adult Mental Health Services & Consultant Clinical Psychologist, South West London and St. George's Mental Health NHS Trust, UK

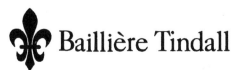

EDINBURGH   LONDON   NEW YORK   OXFORD   PHILADELPHIA   ST LOUIS   SYDNEY   TORONTO   2003

BAILLIÈRE TINDALL
An imprint of Elsevier Limited

First published 2003
   Reprinted 2004, 2006

ISBN 0 7020 2601 8

British Library Cataloguing in Publication Data
A catalogue record for this book is available from the British Library

Library of Congress Cataloguing in Publication Data
A catalogue record for this book is available from the Library of Congress

Note
Medical knowledge is constantly changing. Standard safety precautions must be followed, but as new research and clinical experience broaden our knowledge, changes in treatment and drug therapy may become necessary or appropriate. Readers are advised to check the most current product information provided by the manufacturer of each drug to be administered to verify the recommended dose, the method and duration of administration, and contraindications. It is the responsibility of the practitioner, relying on experience and knowledge of the patient, to determine dosages and the best treatment for each individual patient. Neither the Publisher nor the author assumes any liability for any injury and/or damage to persons or property arising from this publication.

The Publisher

 your source for books,
journals and multimedia
in the health sciences

www.elsevierhealth.com

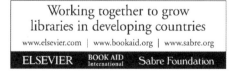

Working together to grow
libraries in developing countries

www.elsevier.com | www.bookaid.org | www.sabre.org

ELSEVIER   BOOK AID International   Sabre Foundation

The publisher's policy is to use **paper manufactured from sustainable forests**

Printed in China
N/03

Contents

Preface

Preface

Every culture recognises in some way the boundaries of 'sanity' and embraces some concept of 'madness' for those who transgress these limits (Murphy 1976, World Health Organisation 1973, 1979, Chadwick 1997a). The situation of those deemed 'mad' has been explained within a variety of religious, spiritual and medical frameworks. As Foucault (1967) argues, 'madness' is treated and constructed in line with the preoccupations of the age. And the way in which 'madness' is constructed determines the value attached to those deemed 'mad', and the options available to them.

The consequences of a label of 'madness' have varied across time and culture (Sayce 2000). Warner (1985) has demonstrated that the outcomes for those who have a diagnosis of schizophrenia are better in 'developing' countries than in the 'developed' world of Europe and North America. In 'developing' countries, madness does not necessarily carry with it the loss of status and exclusion from work and social roles that is the norm in the 'developed' world. Unlike the highly individualised concepts of 'treatment' that prevail in Europe and North America, the rituals and healing ceremonies of some African, Native American and Lapland cultures involve the whole community.

Tempting as it may be to idealise the approaches to 'madness' of other times and places, not all are as humane and inclusive as others (Sayce 2000). For example, while 'village idiots' may have been accepted, they were certainly not valued: Christian notions of 'madness' of the time were linked to sin and possession by the devil. In some African societies, like Zimbabwe, 'madness' is believed to be a consequence of witchcraft – 'ngozi' – and seen as a punishment for wrongdoing by ancestral spirits. Those affected are therefore feared and denigrated. While some native American peoples may have practised healing ceremonies, in others the treatment of those deemed 'mad' was less humane. For example, when one of the wives of a 19th century Pahvant Chief in Utah became insane, according to custom she was tied to a wild horse and dragged to her death (cited in Sayce 2000).

In modern Europe and North America, madness is generally understood in terms of 'illness' and 'brain disease'. Because they are seen as 'ill', people are relieved of their usual roles and responsibilities and their support becomes the province of 'illness' experts: the doctors, nurses, and other therapists who inhabit mental health services. 'Mental illness' is typically defined by these 'experts', most of whom have never experienced that which they seek to describe. The 'mentally ill' are seen as 'other' – a distinct class of person, different and apart from 'normal' people. 'They' become the 'illness' that they are deemed to have – schizophrenics, manic depressives, anorexics – and are deprived of all identities other than that of 'mental patient'. The deficits and dysfunctions that define 'mental illness' provide the justification for their exclusion from the warp and weft of everyday life.

If madness is understood as 'illness' then treatment and cure become the paramount concerns. Although the pharmacological approaches of an organic model remain the most widely used interventions, these are increasingly complemented by a range of psychological and social explanations and their associated therapeutic methodologies. However, these alternative approaches – whether they be organic, psychological, interpersonal or systemic – retain a focus on problems and the ways in which the underlying mechanisms may be addressed to alleviate them. In recognition of the range of supposed underlying mechanisms, it has become popular to talk of 'mental health problems' rather than 'mental illness'. But this semantic shift continues to betray an understanding grounded in notions of treatment and cure (Perkins & Repper 1998). What is a 'health problem' if it is not an 'illness'? We have spent many hours debating the most appropriate language with which to describe those experiences that have been labelled has 'mental illness' (see Perkins & Repper 2001). The language we use is important: it defines the meaning and value of that which is labelled. We might have preferred the term 'madness', but we are aware that this is considered offensive by some people. Therefore, cognizant of its limitations and inaccuracies, we have largely resorted to the commonly used phrase 'mental health problems'.

It is our contention that any approach that focuses on deficit and dysfunction necessarily limits our view of people who experience mental health problems and the possibilities available to them. We are not suggesting that all existing treatments and supports be abandoned, but we would argue that the range of organic, psychological and interpersonal models on which they are based do not constitute an adequate organising principle for understanding the experience of mental health problems or for helping people who experience them. Everyone is more than the sum of his/her problems. And a focus on problems tends to obscure all other facets of the person and their life, suggesting that if these problems can be reduced everything will somehow revert to 'normal'. We know that this is not the case. People whose symptoms continue or recur can, and do, live satisfying lives and contribute to their communities in many different ways, and the alleviation of such symptoms does not necessarily result in the reinstatement of former, valued, roles and relationships.

The specific cognitive and emotional difficulties that led to a diagnosis of mental health problems are usually less disabling than the discrimination and exclusion that accompany them. It is not usually periodic crises or the continuing 'hearing of voices' or 'delusional ideas' that prevent a person from working, studying, or engaging in social and leisure activities. The major barriers lie in prejudice; the belief that anyone who experiences such things cannot possibly do the things that 'normal' people do.

The challenge facing people with mental health problems is to retain, or rebuild, a meaningful and valued life, and, like everyone else, to grow and develop within and beyond the limits imposed by their cognitive and emotional difficulties. Recovery is not about 'getting rid' of problems. It is about seeing people beyond their problems – their abilities, possibilities, interests and dreams – and recovering the social roles and relationships that give life value and meaning. This requires hope and opportunity. Building for a future necessitates a belief in the possibility of that future. Hope is the motivating force that gives life purpose and direction, but, without the opportunity to do the things you want to do, such hope is easily snuffed out.

In this book, we draw on the accounts of people who have themselves faced the challenge of life with a mental health problem, in order to propose that the guiding principles of mental health practice should revolve around social inclusion and recovery. This would involve fostering the hope that is necessary if people are to move beyond mere survival and to thrive, and enabling people to access those activities and relationships that give their lives meaning.

Within these guiding principles, a range of different interventions and supports may be appropriate to different people. A range of therapeutic interventions may be helpful, as might practical help to access opportunities and hope-inspiring relationships. However, if mental health services are to enable people to pursue their aspirations, the key questions must be as follows: do they facilitate the recovery of a meaningful and satisfying life, and do they enable people to do the things they want to do? There can be no set formula. Everyone's journey is different. Traditional yardsticks of success – the alleviation of symptoms and discharge from services – are replaced by questions about whether people are able to do the things that give their lives meaning and purpose, irrespective of whether their problems continue and whether or not they continue to need help and support.

In writing this book we have drawn on our collective experience of over 40 years working within mental health services and over 15 years of personal experience of living with mental health problems. We first met each other two decades ago as newly qualified mental health professionals – Julie a nurse, and Rachel a clinical psychologist – working in a South London rehabilitation service. After leaving clinical practice, Julie worked as a lecturer in nursing studies and as a researcher, and is now employed as a Senior Research Fellow at the University of Sheffield and Lead Research Nurse with Community Health Sheffield NHS Trust. In addition to her involvement in a range of research and service-development work, she has a particular interest

in promoting user-led research initiatives. After 20 years working within reha-
bilitation services, as both a clinician and Clinical Director, Rachel is now the
Clinical Director of Adult Mental Health Services at South West London and
St George's Mental Health NHS Trust, and is a specialist adviser with the
Health Advisory Service. She has a particular interest in disability rights and
employment and mental health, and established the 'Pathfinder User
Employment Programme', an initiative designed to increase access within
mental health services for people who have themselves experienced mental
health problems. In addition to our 'day jobs', Julie is a Trustee of Nottingham
Advocacy Group and a member of the Board of Governors at the school that
her daughters attend, and, in this capacity, has participated in a 'mental
health and emotional well-being' campaign at the school. Rachel is a member
of the Council of the Manic Depression Fellowship and Mental Health Media,
and a member of the Mental Health Action Group of the Disability Rights
Commission.

This is the third book that we have written together. [Our two previous
jointly authored books were *Working Alongside People with Long Term Mental
Health Problems* (Perkins & Repper 1996) and *Dilemmas in Community Mental
Health Practice. Choice or Control* (Perkins & Repper 1998).] It was born of 20
years of shared argument and debate, joint and separate work, and living with
our own mental health problems. This book is written for all those working
in statutory and voluntary mental health services. The ideas we present may
be considered controversial by some, but we hope that they will, at the very
least, provoke thought and debate. We start from the belief that people with
mental health problems have a right to participate, as equal citizens, in all the
opportunities available within the communities of their choice. As mental
health workers we need to move away from a perspective that considers
'patients in our services' to one of serving people in their communities,
enabling people to live the lives they wish to lead.

In writing this book we owe a great deal to many people. We cannot name
them all here, but we would like to say a special 'thank you' to Liz Sayce and
Dean Repper for helping us to refine our ideas, and to Peter Bates for his *A–Z
of Strategies for Social Inclusion*. Most of all, we would like to thank the many
people with mental health problems whom we have had the privilege to
know, both personally and through their writing. More than all our degrees
and professional qualifications, it is these people who have been our most
powerful inspiration and our most influential guides.

Rachel Perkins
Julie Repper
May 2002

Section 1

Recovery: the expertise of experience

1

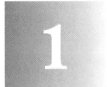

Another way: beyond symptoms and deficits

INTRODUCTION

Schizophrenia, manic depression, depression, anxiety and all other categories of mental health problems developed by professionals are defined in terms of clusters of symptoms. Diagnoses are made on the basis of symptoms such as 'delusional beliefs', 'auditory hallucinations', 'ideas of reference', 'pressure of speech', 'flight of ideas', and 'suicidal ideation', or, in more psychological terms, phenomena such as 'thinking errors' like 'selective abstraction' or 'over-generalisation' and 'defence mechanisms' such as 'denial' or 'projection'. It is in terms of such symptoms that professionals seek to understand the experience of 'madness'.

Evidence of a person's symptoms is sought in the descriptions they provide of thoughts, feelings and behaviour. So, for example, when Beverley said that she was a member of the royal family, and that she knew this because of the way in which her name is spelt, she was deemed to have 'delusional beliefs' and was accorded a diagnosis of schizophrenia. While diagnosis may provide a way of naming distress and disability, this symptom-based description tells us little about the person's life and experience. No-one made any effort to explore Beverley's beliefs fully, because they felt that it would be bad for her. They believed that to 'collude with a delusion' would only reinforce that delusion. Beverley therefore became angry and complained that staff 'wouldn't listen to her' and 'didn't understand'.

Yet listening to what Beverley had to say revealed that she believed she had been thrown out of the royal household when she was a baby because she was black. She thought that, because black people are inferior in England, the royal family could not have had a black baby in its midst and, therefore, at an early age she had been put up for adoption by her true parents and brought up by a black family. She was angry that she had been denied the status, privileges and respect that were due to her as a member of the royal family, and so repeatedly wrote to the Queen (whom she believed to be her aunt) at Buckingham Palace, asking for her help.

It is likely that few people would share Beverley's understanding of her situation. It is easy to write off her beliefs as false. Whilst we may doubt their accuracy in literal terms, these beliefs take on a different meaning in the light of her life and experience. Beverley's parents came from Jamaica, but she was born in England. In the largely white area where she lived, she experienced a great deal of racism. She always felt like an outsider and dreamed of what she saw as her real home in Jamaica. When she was in her early teens she finally went to visit this 'home', but actually felt just as much of an outsider among her relatives in Jamaica as she had done in England. She retained a feeling of 'not belonging' and 'not being wanted' that was reinforced by later events. When she was 16 she had a boyfriend of whom her parents did not approve. She left the family home to live with him. Shortly after her child was born, her partner became extremely violent towards her and for several years she frequently left him for the safety of a refuge for women who had experienced domestic violence. But, when accused of stealing from other women in the refuge, this escape route was denied her. Having no resources and nowhere to go, she was arrested for theft, and, after spending a short time in prison, was admitted to a psychiatric hospital. She was eventually discharged to a hostel, but the placement didn't last long: she apparently refused to take part in the life of the hostel (sharing in the cleaning, cooking of meals, etc.) and frequently became angry and threatening towards other residents because she believed that they looked down on her. After a series of admissions she had nowhere to go but the psychiatric hospital. By this time she had lost all her friends and family, she had only her 'hospital pocket money' on which to live, and her frequently hostile behaviour made her unpopular among both staff and other residents.

In order to begin to understand and help Beverley it is not enough to see her simply as someone with 'delusional beliefs' and 'treatment-resistant schizophrenia': the belief that one is really a member of the royal family takes on a different meaning in the context of her life. If you have lost everything, never felt that you belong anywhere, repeatedly been devalued and rejected, then the belief that you are a member of the royal family – someone worthy of respect and dignity – is perhaps understandable. In helping her, restoring dignity and self-respect was at least as important as treating her symptomatology.

SYMPTOMS: A FAINT ECHO OF EXPERIENCE

The gulf between lived experiences and the accounts of mental health professionals can be immense. O'Hagan (1996) illustrates this divide by putting together notes from her own diary with those from her medical file, both written during an in-patient admission. For example, on one day she wrote in her diary:

> *Today I wanted to die. Everything was hurting. My body was screaming.*
> *I saw the doctor. I said nothing. Now I feel terrible. Nothing seems good*
> *and nothing good seems possible.*
> *   I am stuck in this twilight mood*
> *Where I go down*
> *Like the setting sun*
> *Into a lonely black hole*
> *Where there is room for only one.*

At the same time, her hospital file reported:

> *Flat. Lacking in motivation, sleep and appetite good. Discussed aetiology.*
> *Cont. LiCarb 250 mg qid. Levels next time.*

A similar contrast is illustrated by Alexander (1994):

> *The hospital record stated: 'Patient slowly staggered to the end of the*
> *hall, but did not write anything'. My own account reads: 'At the last safe*
> *table, I'm pushed and placed into the last safe chair. All the universe is*
> *compacted into this four square table of suffering wood. On the table lies*
> *a piece of metal, glimmering. It's my Saviour friend – all that's left of*
> *him after he's suffered through the endless rounds of the Hitler machine.'*
> *The story ended with me being given a pen and paper to write the 'last*
> *page of history'. But I couldn't write because black ink meant it would*
> *end in death.*
> *   Psychiatry could read this as a paranoid delusion, yet to me the*
> *glimmering bit of metal offered hope.*

Numerous personal accounts of the experience of mental health problems are now available, and they offer insights that can never be gained from symptomatic and diagnostic descriptions:

> *On Saturday I woke at dawn and left the house within an hour. I felt*
> *tremendous. Things had finally slotted into place and I was going to*
> *convert the 'natives' of the Upper Niger, equipped only with inspiration*
> *and a portable gramophone. Two hours later I tried to cross the*
> *Broadway opposite Hammersmith Odeon with my eyes closed. I laid my*
> *possessions outside the door to the church by the flyover and built a*
> *diagrammatic Calvary on the path. (Campbell 1996a)*

> *One night during my freshman year at college, I stepped out of the dorm,*
> *intending never to return … A symbolic word started to erupt as I*
> *wandered on campus. When a stranger asked for directions, I feared he*

had a gun – that he was <u>Death.</u> I responded 'I'm new here.' Somehow, it was true, I felt – <u>I was new here.</u> It was raining and cold as I walked into the countryside. The irrationality of going out alone into the night, intending to leave all behind – even my family – awoke deep feelings of sadness in me. But I had to continue on. I felt a <u>test</u> from the sky: to walk all night without stopping or resting … The <u>tests</u> felt as if <u>they came from outside,</u> as a demand from the universe … To me it wasn't a 'delusion' implying falsity and blockage … When dawn came, I had clearly entered the symbolic world. Colors were swirling, <u>matter was rising to life.</u> A train passed by, encircling me faster and faster. 'The Morning Trains have risen,' I thought, 'but no one is guiding them.' (Alexander 1994)

Haze and fog are often used to describe depression. However, it seems appropriate to describe both the emotional and cognitive blunting as semi-existence within the interior of a marshmallow. (Berman 1994)

The double reality … was being maintained – at one stratum events occurred which seemed quite innocent and innocuous, but on another level they had a portentous and sinister meaning directed at me, all in the service of driving me to self-destruction. It was like a Euripidean dual-plane Greek tragedy: the gods above, at one level of meaning, everyday life below, at another, transferred to the latter half of the twentieth century. (Chadwick 1997b)

Forming a relationship with someone whose experience of reality is profoundly different from your own is not easy. In describing his experience of hospitalisation with a diagnosis of schizophrenia Chadwick (1997b) cautions:

… when dealing with a newly admitted deluded patient the terms on which you think the interaction is taking place are not anything like the terms as seen from the patient's perspective. It is not simply a matter of there being likely suspiciousness, misinterpretation, and misunderstanding, the patient is literally living and behaving in a different world from you. The 'plane of meaning' that you are tuned into is markedly oblique to theirs.

However, it would be a mistake to assume that everything a person says or does is always framed within this 'other' world. It is very easy to write off everything as being related only to the person's 'delusional' ideas, but such an error has resulted in a great many of the complaints of service users being discounted as symptoms of their 'madness'. As Nicola Padgett put it:

Madness is very specific. When you think that the first piece of loo paper is poisoned, you also know that you have a relaxation class at half past two. So you know what a relaxation class is, and what half past two is. (cited in Brooks 1997)

Any therapeutic relationship which really enables a person to grow and develop must be based on understanding: an understanding not only of a person's life and experiences more generally, but of their experience of 'symptoms'. This can never be furnished by a diagnosis and list of symptoms alone: 'outer symptoms are but a faint echo of the inner process' (Alexander 1994).

DEFICITS OR POSSIBILITIES?

Probably because the experience of 'madness' is traditionally described by those who have never experienced it, the phenomena associated with it are invariably seen in negative terms, i.e. as shortcomings, deficits and distortions.

> "... even the briefest perusal of the current literature on schizophrenia will immediately reveal to the uninitiated that this collection of problems is viewed by practitioners almost exclusively in terms of dysfunction and disorder. A positive or charitable phrase or sentence rarely meets the eye..." (Chadwick 1997b).

Having defined conditions such as schizophrenia as 'disorders', most research proceeds to identify the deficits manifested by people with this disorder: the mental health literature is replete with studies of this kind (see, for example, Cutting & Murphy 1988, Morice 1990, Morice & Delahunty 1996).

There is no doubt that the experience of mental health problems is, for many people, a distressing and debilitating one. However, in his book *Schizophrenia: The Positive Perspective*, Chadwick (1997b) describes the shortcomings of research based on the quest for deficits. First, he argues that this severely colours the attitudes of mental health workers, particularly their perception of the dignity of their clients.

> *Deficit-obsessed research can only produce theories and attitudes which are disrespectful of clients and are also likely to induce behaviour in clinicians such that service users are not properly listened to, not believed, not fairly assessed, are likely treated as inadequate and are also not expected to be able to become independent and competent individuals in managing life's tasks.* (Chadwick 1997b)

He argues that such a focus on the part of professionals and researchers shapes the prevailing construction of 'madness' as a wholly negative phenomenon, inevitably contributing to negative public attitudes towards people with mental health problems.

Second, he argues that a continual focus on the negative has a destructive impact on the person who experiences mental health problems: 'Forever harping on disasters, dangers, deficits and dysfunctions does not encourage the strength needed to overcome the problems that present themselves.'

(Chadwick 1997b). Such an approach can eradicate any hope that recovery is even a possibility, and without hope there can appear to be little point in trying to overcome difficulties.

Third, he argues that a full understanding of the nature of 'disorders' such as schizophrenia and manic depression must include a quest for 'schizophrenic credit' (Claridge 1985) – those areas of functioning in which the psychosis-prone mind might be <u>better</u> than that of 'standard-minded' people. It is a mistake always to look for meaning in the extremes of experience: he argues that a more fertile ground for understanding the real nature of the condition lies in the 'transition zone' – the borderlands between sanity and insanity. He cites advantages such as greater empathy and creativity – sometimes labelled 'superphrenic' (Karlsson, 1972) – which may be associated with 'disorders' such as schizophrenia. Similarly, Jamison (1989, 1993, 1995a,b) has described evidence which shows a relationship between creativity and mood disorders.

There are numerous descriptions of famous artists, writers, scientists, and leaders who have experienced mental health problems. Post (1994, 1996), in his work on psychopathology and creativity, cites hundreds of famous people (including statesmen like Parnell, scientists like Einstein and Babbage, scholars like Wittgenstein and Ruskin, composers like Ravel, visual artists like Van Gogh, and novelists like Auden and Chesterton) with paranoid, schizoid and schizotypal traits.

Jamison (1995a), an eminent academic and researcher, describes her own experiences of manic depression. Although these have been distressing and debilitating, they have also been positive and creative: 'The ideas and feelings are fast and furious like shooting stars ... shyness goes, the right words are suddenly there, the power to captivate others a felt certainty.' Similarly, Lawrence (1998) cites 75 great men and women whom, he argues, have achieved their greatness not in spite of their manic depression, but because of it. These include Bach, Churchill, Handel, Keats, Roosevelt, Tolstoy, Wagner and Wolf. He offers a description of his own manic depression – and that of others – which is in marked contrast to the gloomy picture presented by many mental health professionals:

> *From suicidal subsistence, in the pits of the darkest despair (stage 1),*
> *a mood can elevate to normal (stage 2), like a lift at street-level, with*
> *communication to the world outside. Rising still further, the manic can put*
> *head and shoulders above the crowd, with merriment and inventiveness.*
> *This third stage is that of Hypomania, in which genius, if present, begins to*
> *be manifest. Seemingly, genius operates by the unusual development of*
> *lateral and multilateral thinking, giving rise to mild eccentricities,*
> *parodies, inspirations. Sometimes shafts of brilliant light may be departed*

from the traces of creativity kicked over. Stage four is Mania itself, a wild, flamboyant rushing of ideas, turbulently juggling in a cranium too cramped to cope. Some exciting paintings, symphonies, phrases and phases of scientific invention may have composed themselves in minds experiencing the fires of Mania.

Even distressing and debilitating experiences do not have to be cast in purely negative terms. Barker et al, (1999) provide a number of first-person accounts in which the occurrence of mental health problems offered an opportunity for development and growth. Others echo the benefits they have gained from frightening and disabling experiences:

I have often asked myself whether, given the choice, I would choose to have manic depressive illness.... Strangely enough I think I would choose to have it. It's complicated. Depression is awful beyond words or sounds or images ... So why would I want anything to do with this illness? Because I honestly believe that as a result of it I have felt more things, more deeply; had more experiences, more intensely; loved more, and been loved; laughed more often for having cried more often; appreciated more the springs, for all the winters; worn death 'as close as dungarees', appreciated it – and life – more; seen the finest and the most terrible in people, and slowly learned the values of caring, loyalty and seeing things through. (Jamison 1995a)

As I found myself, psychosis – particularly in the early euphoric phase, if it obtains – can be at least the beginning of spiritual enlightenment. It may open doors to such experiences that the person can make productive use of later when they are well. (Chadwick 1997b)

Because I have faced this pain, I am able to feel more deeply, reach out to others more authentically. To this day, the experience's bewildering array of symbolism involves me in its interpretation. Much of it involved the modern day anxiety toward death: from the stranger who I first met who I thought was death, to the attempt to write the last page of history in black. But the experience also showed me that there is a world on the other side of death. (Alexander 1994)

For many, the experience of mental distress and disability is undoubtedly awful and debilitating. Many fail to accommodate it within their lives. Lawrence (1998) speculates: 'Are their intellects too frail to channel the lava flow or have they not found a media in which to cast it?' Yet it is impossible to believe that the negative way in which mental health problems are typically viewed does not have a destructive impact on those who experience them. If you are faced by a world that regards those with mental health problems as incompetent (Ridgeway 1988), it is difficult to continue to believe in yourself and see anything positive in your experiences. This is compounded if mental health workers echo these popular beliefs. Strauss (1985) makes a direct link between the negative messages that people are given and their 'demoralisation':

> *Some of the most common treatment efforts may inadvertently create the opposite effect from the one intended. Patients with schizophrenia are often told they have a disease like diabetes. They are told that they will have the disease all their lives, that it involves major and permanent functional impairment and they will have a life long need for medication.... Withdrawal, that is to say isolation and alienation and the associated phenomena of amotivation, apathy, and anhedonia, are partly a manifestation of demoralisation. Indeed, much of what has been described as the 'negative symptom syndrome' is attributable to demoralisation ...*

How many times have clients heard the 'you'll nevers' from professionals determined to be 'realistic': 'You'll never lead an ordinary life again', 'You have difficulties looking after yourself, you'll never be able to have children', 'You'll never be able to go back to your job', and so on? For example, research indicates that 44% of those people with mental health problems who had been successful in gaining employment had been told by a mental health worker that they would never work again (Rinaldi 2000). How many times do mental health workers encourage those whom they serve to see the positive possibilities for life with mental health problems? How often do we cite examples of the achievements of those who have experienced such difficulties?

A vicious cycle of incompetence is all too easily established. If we see mental health problems solely in terms of deficits and dysfunctions, we define those who experience them as incompetent. This means that people have two options. One option is to accept the professionals' bleak prophecies, define themselves in those terms, and give up. They will cease to use their skills and lose many through lack of use, thus reinforcing their own, and others', views of their incompetency. Alternatively, they can reject professionals' gloomy prognoses, reject the services that deem them incompetent, and hence fail to receive the support they might need in order to make the most of their lives.

Perhaps it is difficult for mental health workers to see the other side of the coin – people who have mental health problems living meaningful, fulfilling and productive lives – because they only see people when their problems are at their worst. When problems subside, people tend to move away from services – to a place where they cannot easily be seen by mental health workers.

Mental health workers tend to get a very negative view of people with psychosis as they usually only see people when they are most disturbed. They don't see the ones like me who got away. Therefore they have very little concept of recovery from mental health problems or the positive aspects of madness. (May, cited in British Psychological Society 2000)

Deficit and dysfunction are part of the story – but only a part of it. If we are to help those who experience mental health problems we must be able to see the positive possibilities open to them.

MORE THAN REDUCING SYMPTOMS AND PROBLEMS . . .

A focus on deficits and dysfunctions has led to services whose primary aim is to reduce such symptoms and problems. We assess need in terms of symptoms to be alleviated, focus interventions on difficulties, and evaluate effectiveness in terms of symptom removal ('cure'). Such an approach is not limited to doctors or to an 'organic' perspective. Most mental health workers begin by defining deficits and then direct their endeavours, and evaluate their success, in terms of the extent to which these problems have been removed. We might, for example, decide that a person has deficits in self-care, or difficulties using community facilities, or problems in relating to other people, and direct our attentions to improving these aspects.

How different would our services look if their primary focus was to enable people to use and develop their skills, make the most of their assets and pursue their aspirations? Would this not change, for the better, the experience of using services, and the relationships between workers and those whom we serve?

While people with mental health problems may desire freedom from debilitating symptoms, this is only part of the story: they typically place at least as much emphasis on the importance of decent lives:

. . . safe, pleasant and affordable housing, well paying and fulfilling jobs . . . to be treated with dignity and respect, to have control over their lives and to have genuine choices. They want to feel good about themselves and to have the opportunity to achieve things that all of us do. (Bond 1994)

Shepherd et al (1995) found differences in the priorities of mental health workers and those who use their services. Clients valued help in coming to terms with their problems, together with assistance with housing, finance, social networks and physical health, while workers placed greater emphasis on professional support, treatment and monitoring. More recently, user-led research conducted by the Mental Health Foundation (Faulkner & Layzell

2000) found a series of common themes in what people sought from services; the removal of symptoms was notably absent from their list, which comprised the following items:

◆ acceptance
◆ shared experience – shared identity: the company of others who shared similar experiences
◆ emotional support – 'being there'
◆ a reason for living
◆ finding meaning and purpose in their lives
◆ peace of mind and relaxation
◆ taking control and having choices
◆ security and safety
◆ pleasure.

If we are to develop services that reflect the goals of those who use them, then we must listen to what they have to say. As mental health workers we must broaden our horizons. Living with mental health problems involves a great deal more than symptom control. We must examine the extent to which what we do enables people to achieve their own goals, and accept that symptom reduction does not necessarily improve quality of life:

> *the assumption that symptom relief, reduction in the frequency of episodes of illness and improvement in functional adaptation ... mean that quality of life has been enhanced may at times be unwarranted. Indeed, for some patients, these seemingly positive changes may not be accompanied by the development of meaningful interpersonal relationships, by employment that they are enthusiastic about, or by a subjective sense of satisfaction and well-being ... Emphasis should be placed not only on level of clinical symptomatology or pathologic behaviour, but also on the functional integration of the patient into his occupational, social and cultural milieu.* (Mirin & Namerow 1991)

There is also no necessary connection between a reduction in symptom severity and a person's sense of control or engagement. For example, vocational rehabilitation research has failed to demonstrate a relationship between diagnosis or symptom severity and employment (e.g. Anthony et al 1995). Similarly, Strauss (1994) has described how, with effective support, those whose symptoms do not improve may still report an increased sense of control, or increased understanding of their problems, which is associated with a reduction in distress and despair.

In our professional quest to remove people's symptoms and problems it is easy to forget that they have lives to lead. Mental health problems are not a full-time occupation, but they can too easily take over the whole of your life. In order to prevent this happening, it is essential that mental health workers move beyond the narrow goals of symptom relief and problem reduction. If everyone concentrates on what you <u>cannot</u> do, then it is easy to lose confidence in yourself as a worthwhile person and lose sight of life's possibilities. Mental health services are replete with people who have 'given up' on themselves and their futures – a tragic waste of human lives and potential.

Mental health workers are clearly in a powerful position with respect to the people who use their services. Such power, in part, derives from mental health legislation, but it also arises from the power of expertise and status. And such power must be used sensitively.

RECOGNITION OF DIFFERENCE

Professionals define the nature and implications of mental health problems not only for the individual concerned, but within the wider society. They have a great deal of direct and indirect power in determining people's future possibilities. If the 'experts' tell you that you are able, or not able, to do things, then you are more likely to believe them than if you were told the same things by your next-door neighbour. If the 'experts' say that people with mental health problems are dangerous and unpredictable, then this will influence the way in which they are understood and treated in the wider society. Employers, neighbours, and providers of goods and services are influenced by 'expert' opinions which therefore determine the opportunities available to people with mental health problems.

While this situation raises important questions about the relative status of different sorts of expertise – the expertise of personal experience versus the expertise of degrees and qualifications – the reality is that these power differentials do exist. Professionals must therefore be aware of the implications of what they say at all levels: whether they are talking about the nature of mental health difficulties or to people who are experiencing them.

Most professionals do not know what life with a mental health problem is like. It is important, therefore, that we recognise the limits of our expertise. Many of us will not have experienced the myriad difficulties with which some people have to contend: racism, sexism, heterosexism, poverty, exclusion from school, disrupted family life, domestic violence, sexual abuse, being a refugee or asylum seeker, etc. The critical thing is that, as mental health workers, we acknowledge and respect these differences, accept our own limitations, and recognise the wisdom endowed by first-hand experience. People can gain a great deal of support, information and hope – a vision of the possible – from those who have faced similar challenges.

VALUING THE EXPERTISE OF EXPERIENCE

Increasing numbers of service-users are recognising the limitations of professional expertise:

> *Ex-patients ... are beginning to turn to each other rather than to mental health professionals for emotional and instrumental support. They are finding that people with experiential knowledge (i.e. having learned through personal experience) are more able to understand their needs than are professionals who have learned through education and training. Moreover, they are finding the support and help they can give each other to be as valuable – or sometimes more valuable – than the interventions of trained professionals.* (Wilson Besio 1987)

'They never listen' is one of the most persistent complaints of people who use mental health services (Lindow 1996). Their words are too often heard only in order to diagnose.

> *I can talk, but I may not be heard. I can make suggestions, but they may not be taken seriously. I can voice my thoughts, but they may be seen as delusions. I can recite my experiences, but they may be interpreted as fantasies. To be an ex-patient or even an ex-client is to be discounted.* (Leete 1988a)

In moving beyond symptoms and deficits, it is vital that we start in a different place, i.e. with the voice of first-hand experience. We need to begin by listening to people who have mental health problems. We must gain insight into the possibilities of life with mental health problems. Mental health workers often place great emphasis on promoting insight in patients (Kemp et al 1996). Perhaps we should pay more attention to mental health workers' insight into the experiences, challenges, aspirations and lives of those who use our services.

2

To be a mental patient: the nature of the challenge

INTRODUCTION

In a social context in which being a mental patient means being devalued and excluded – considered unpredictable, dangerous, incapable of living an ordinary life – it is hardly surprising that people find being diagnosed as 'mentally ill' devastating.

> *When I was diagnosed I felt this is the end of my life. It was a thing to isolate me from other human beings. I felt I was not viable unless they found a cure... I felt flawed. Defective.* (cited in Sayce 2000)

> *I yelled at them when they came to see me. I yelled for some time. I really did not want to hear what my two best friends had to say. They told me they thought there was something wrong with me. The sort of something that meant I should see a psychiatrist... You do not decide to become a psychiatric patient: apply for the position as you might for a job, or elect to join as you might a campaigning group. There are no guidelines about how to be a recipient of mental health services. Noone tells you the rules as in a job description... I found myself completely at sea not really knowing what to do and feeling very alone.* (Perkins 1999)

> *Well my mental health started when I was 15 and at school. I wanted to get on and do things, but this stopped me doing it, this mental health... I thought I wanted to be a nurse. Or in the police force. But I didn't get that far. I felt strange. I couldn't cope with things. I got frustrated, angry... I had to stop work... I couldn't cope with life in general... I wanted to end my life.* (cited in Repper et al 1998)

> *They said I would never get better. I would always be mentally ill. They said I would be in and out of mental hospitals the rest of my life.*

I could never be the person I was before my mental illness. (Schmook 1994)

Deegan (1988) draws parallels with a friend who had broken his neck:

At a young age we had both experienced a catastrophic shattering of our world, hopes, and dreams. He had broken his neck and was paralyzed and I was diagnosed as being schizophrenic ... He was an athlete and had dreamed of becoming a professional in the sports world. I was a high school athlete and had applied to college to become a gym teacher. Just days earlier we knew ourselves as young people with exciting futures, and then everything collapsed around us. As teenagers we were told we would be 'sick' or 'disabled' for the rest of our lives.

O'Donoghue (1994) has listed common responses to diagnosis:

◆ Shame: 'Oh dear, I hope no one finds out.'
◆ Terror: 'Now what will happen to me?'
◆ Isolation: 'No one will want to know me.'
◆ Grief: 'My life is over.'
◆ Mistake: 'It must be a mistake.'
◆ Anger: 'Why me? It's not fair.'

To these might be added guilt ('I must have done something very wrong.'), worthlessness ('Everyone else manages, I'm just not good enough.'), hopelessness ('There's no point in carrying on.'), despair, giving up ...

Many of these responses will have a familiar ring to them. They are all characteristic of a grieving process. Kubler-Ross (1969) has described the stages that people go through in order to cope with a loss or bereavement. These stages do not necessarily occur in consecutive order, but they must take place in order for grief to be resolved; recovery cannot begin until the loss has been accepted. The stages are outlined below.

◆ Denial: 'No, not me', 'it must be a mistake.', 'it's not happening to me.', 'Everything will be back to normal soon.' Disbelief and shock permit the person to develop ways of coping with the reality of the loss.
◆ Anger: 'Why me?' Resentment and blame are directed towards family members, healthcare staff, God ....
◆ Bargaining: 'Give me another year and I'll ...'. The individual vows to live life in a different way if the loss can be ameliorated in some way.
◆ Depression: 'Yes me.' The individual acknowledges the reality of the situation, which brings sadness, hopelessness and despair.
◆ Acceptance: The individual experiences the pain of the loss, adjusts to the new world without the lost 'object', and reinvests in a new way of life.

If to have mental health problems is to be seen as defective, then it is hardly surprising that many reject this definition of themselves. Sometimes such denial is seen as pathological, i.e. inherent in the 'illness' itself – a manifestation of 'lack of insight'. However, it can also be seen as an adaptive coping strategy:

> *... we didn't believe our doctors and social workers. In fact, we adamantly denied and raged against these bleak prophecies for our lives. We felt it was just all a mistake, a bad dream ... in a week or two things would be back to normal again ... Our denial was an important stage in our recovery. It was a normal reaction to an overwhelming situation. It was our way of surviving those first awful months.* (Deegan 1988)

Denial of devastating life events is certainly not restricted to mental illness. Such disbelief is often the initial response to any bereavement, for example when your partner leaves, when someone you love dies, when you find a lump in your breast, when you fail a critical examination, and so on.

Denial and disbelief are often closely followed by anger.

> *Anger follows on the footsteps of despair and grieving. Anger at the illness which has so devastated us. Anger at the helping system which may have failed and even bruised us at times. Anger at society and its attitudes. Anger at God for not taking better care of us. Anger at parents and friends for not being more helpful. Anger at ourself for not being able to manage our illness. Our anger is a necessary and important part of the process. Anger is a stimulus to recovery. It is normal and natural.* (Spaniol & Koehler 1994)

But anger readily gives way to hopelessness and despair.

> *We both gave up. Giving up was a solution for us. It numbed the pain of our despair ... All of us who have experienced catastrophic illness and disability know this experience of anguish and despair. It is living in darkness without hope, without a past or a future ... It is rage turned inward ... It is ... a death from which there appears no hope of resurrection. It is inertia that paralyzes the will to do and to accomplish, because there is no hope.* (Deegan 1988)

To be diagnosed as having mental health problems is indeed a bereavement: it involves loss of the privileges of sanity, loss of the life we had (or had expected to lead), and loss of the person we had thought we were or might become. This bereavement is disabling in and of itself; it typically takes years to heal the wounds. Yet all too often within mental health services, the bereavement of diagnosis is ignored, eclipsed by a concern with the control of symptoms.

When expressed by people with mental health problems, the ordinary responses to bereavement can be regarded as symptoms of disorder: rage and crying might be interpreted as 'acting out', apathy and withdrawal as 'negative symptoms'.

> *Some people will try to tell you that your anger is a symptom of mental illness. Don't believe them. Anger is not a symptom of mental illness. Some people may even try to medicate you in order to make your anger go away. This can be dangerous – by extinguishing someone's anger we run the risk of breaking their spirit and of wounding their dignity . . . .*
> *Your anger is not a symptom of mental illness. Your angry indignation is a sane response to the situation you are facing.* (Deegan 1993)

If any bereavement is not recognised, and grieving is not allowed to take its course, then the impact of that bereavement is magnified. Without time and space to process what has happened – to find a way through it – the continuing impact of the loss is all the more devastating. The bereavement of diagnosis is no different: 'For some of us this dark night lasts moments, days or months. For others it lasts for years. For others the despair and anguish may never end.' (Deegan 1993).

UNSHARED EXPERIENCES

The isolation and disadvantage that accompany a diagnosis of mental health problems are compounded by the experience of the (often frightening) symptoms on which diagnosis was based. Subsumed under umbrella terms – delusions, flight of ideas, depressed affect – these experiences may be profoundly different from those of other people. It is difficult to explain or understand experiences that are so unlike those of others.

Unless you have experienced it yourself, it is difficult to imagine what it is like to be unable to organise your own thoughts:

> *My thoughts get all jumbled up. I start thinking or talking about something and I never get there. Instead I wander off in the wrong direction and get caught up with all sorts of different things.* (Torrey 1983)

> *My mind is like a pile*
> *of broken up smudgy thoughts.*
> *I am searching for one*
> *That is clear enough to have meaning.*
> *But as soon as I find a thought*
> *It gets sucked into the blackness.* (O'Hagan 1996)

It is also difficult to imagine finding the ordinary things of everyday life impossibly difficult:

To get out of bed at midday was an ordeal. I felt I had nothing to look forward to, no interest in anything – in short, I felt totally apathetic. I couldn't even be bothered to talk to my girlfriend or father, the two people who were closest to me. I had no interests at all. I wouldn't listen to the radio or stereo, or watch TV, never mind go out. I never had the desire to drink beer! ... I would just lie on my bed, staring at the ceiling ... Often I would burst into tears for no apparent reason.
(A Psychiatric Nurse 1996)

Similarly, it is hard to understand what it is like to experience altered sensations and perceptions that no-one else appears to share:

Rachel, they're back, the air bubbles. At first I always believed they were part of every day, then you didn't know what I meant. I realised I was the only one who had them – bubbles hitting me ... from every side, and my head is empty, empty as a shell, all of my thoughts drained out of me while I was asleep. All mixed up, day, night, whispers all around my head, lots of water, shoes don't seem to fit, colours, it's all going on at once – it's killing me. (cited in Kitzinger & Perkins 1993)

Everything hurts.
I am burning.
All the life in me
Blazing out from the core of me
Is getting stuck.
I can feel it
Trying to burn through my skin.
I am almost on fire. (O'Hagan 1996)

It is difficult, too, to imagine how it feels to know that strange things are happening – things that are at odds with what others believe:

I believed the television and radio had interactive messages for me. I also believed I had unknowingly been a spy ... Nothing was as it appeared with robotic surveillance pets and sinister tracking devices. I also saw familiar faces in strangers faces, which lead to further espionage theories. I believed I was in danger of losing my ability to think freely and spontaneously, that I would become an automaton ... (May, cited in British Psychological Society 2000)

It is all too tempting for others to dismiss such events as totally ludicrous, imagined, untrue, to interpret what the person does as being a fault of their laziness, lack of consideration for others, 'lack of motivation' or 'attention seeking', or to deem their actions as irrational and unprovoked. Isolation and distress are often exacerbated by the lack of understanding or the disbelief of others. A great deal of what passes for reassurance is often very far from reassuring, but instead makes the person feel misunderstood and even more alone:

> *It was really exciting when I first heard the messages from NASA. I knew about lots of wicked inventions. I had to tell people about them. My Dad told me I was talking rubbish – he just didn't understand – so I walked all the way to Capital Radio – but they didn't want to know. They didn't believe me. They wouldn't let me in. What was I supposed to do? I don't tell people about them now.*

Cognitive and emotional experiences which no one else shares mean that a person has to balance their own, often scary, internal world, with the world that others know:

> *My world is like having two or more different levels of what is right and what is wrong. Should I be pulling myself out to face the everyday motions of life there in your world? Having to keep it up is very difficult. I want to say slow down, have a rest, yet reality goes on and I feel as if I am being smothered by life itself. My world hurts. It's never ending and painful. When I'm in my world I know I'm going far away, and although I know this, I can't prevent it. To me it's all so real, and I honestly believe it to be true and genuine when I'm there* (cited in Kitzinger & Perkins 1993)

> *Glassy shadows, polished pastels, a jigsaw puzzle of my body, face and clothes with pieces disappearing whenever I move. And if I want to reach out to touch me, I feel nothing but slippery coldness … I know I am a 37 year old woman, a sculptor, a writer, a worker, I live alone. I know all of this, but, like the reflection in the glass, my existence seems undefined – more a mirage that I keep reaching for but never can touch.* (McGrath 1984)

We prefer to use terms like 'unshared perceptions' and 'unusual experiences' instead of the more usual 'delusions' and 'hallucinations'. The latter carry the implicit assumption that the person's beliefs are, by definition, unfounded. But the nature of 'truth' is not absolute. People understand the world in different ways and it is impossible to say which of these are 'true' and which are not. In former times, it was 'true' that the world was flat, that the sun revolved around the earth: those who suggested otherwise were 'mad'. In current times, evidence for the existence of the various deities in which so many believe is as slim as that for the 'delusions' of people with mental health problems. The critical issue is the impact of these beliefs on the person's life. Belief in various deities is, for many people, comforting, constructive, and the basis for growth and development, but it can also be destructive, as demonstrated by the numerous religious conflicts and wars that continue around the world.

Understanding and empathy are critical in the formation of the relationships that underlie all effective help. In order to reach any kind of understanding, mental health workers must be willing to explore the experiences of those with whom they work. However, expression of genuine curiosity and interest may be hampered in three ways.

First, there is our understanding of what it means to be a mental health professional. As practitioners, we often believe that, because of our professional training, we are better able to understand a person's situation than he/she can. We are the experts and we know best. But, unless we acknowledge the expertise that personal experience brings, it is unlikely that we will spend time trying to understand a person's situation from their own perspective.

A related barrier that our notion of professionalism may raise is the belief that we must provide answers rather than ask questions. Thus, Felton (in Repper et al 2001) explains that, as a student nurse, she feels able to 'reveal her ignorance' and ask people about their experiences when they are in a classroom context. Yet, in a service setting, the same individuals are 'the patients'. She sees her role to be about providing that help and support – not learning from them. We would not wish to argue that clinicians have no skills, rather that we do not have a monopoly on expertise: understanding the perspective of another person is essential if we are to be able to put our expertise at the disposal of that individual in a constructive way.

Second, there are the 'them and us' distinctions that underpin prejudice and discrimination and pervade mental health services. People with mental health problems are devalued, and, therefore, those who work with them are also devalued by association: this is termed 'courtesy stigma' (Goffman 1963) or 'stigma by association' (Neuberg et al 1994) ('They must be mad to want to work with them.'; 'What's the point in trying to help them?' 'They can't amount to much anyway.'). The image of a psychiatric nurse, for example, is quite different from that of a life-giving midwife or a life-saving Accident and Emergency sister. In comparison with those working in intensive care, operating theatres and medical wards, psychiatric nurses receive least 'recognition, affirmation, acknowledgement and validation' from their family and friends (Cronin-Stubbs & Brophy 1985).

In order to preserve our status, it can be very tempting for mental health workers to dissociate themselves from devalued 'patients', to amplify differences in order to reduce the perceived threat from 'out-group' members (Heatherton et al 2000). Such differentiation is often unconscious or inadvertent. For example, we may be helping someone to travel on a bus, or use a café, or go to the swimming pool – anywhere where there are other people around. The person is attracting negative attention from others. Perhaps it is the way they look, or perhaps they are behaving in a way which is considered to be inappropriate or embarrassing. It is all too tempting to make it clear that we have not chosen to be with this person, that they are not a friend or relation, that they are a 'patient' and we are just there doing our job.

Third, there is the belief that pervades most mental health work that 'you must never collude with a delusion' (Perkins & Dilks 1992, Perkins & Repper 1996). The origins of this belief are not wholly clear, but many mental health workers continue to defend the view that talking about a person's delusions will reinforce false beliefs and add to their distress and disturbance. At one level, this is intuitively sensible. If someone says something that everyone else knows to be 'untrue', then it is only natural to help them to see the error of their ways. However, it is important to move beyond the intuitive and examine the implications of such an approach. A person whose beliefs are not shared by others will be all too familiar with having them challenged. Most people they meet will have ignored or ridiculed them: 'Don't be silly!', 'That's rubbish!', 'Yes dear, let's have a nice cup of tea.' Denying firmly held beliefs that are important to someone leaves them further isolated – alone in a world that no one else understands or takes seriously.

> *To deny another's reality, to ignore and divert what may be frightening experiences, serves to further isolate them and effectively prevents the formation of a good working relationship. If you knew that you would be arrested if you went outside your house you would expect someone trying to help you to appreciate, empathise with and understand your distress, not ignore or avoid it.* (Perkins & Dilks 1992)

It is possible for us as mental health workers to gain some understanding of people's experiences. It involves accepting that we cannot understand another person's world simply by reference to our own. We need to suspend our disbelief, enter their world, and accept that what other people have to say is important and real for them and essential to our understanding of them. Our behaviours arise from the way in which we understand the world – whether or not we have mental health problems. Actions are only incomprehensible and unpredictable if we do not understand the beliefs and experiences on which they are based.

ILLNESS OR DISABILITY AND INCLUSION?

An illness model is the predominant framework for understanding difficulties with thinking and feeling. This framework has been described as 'the medical model' but might more accurately be labelled an 'organic model'. It is a perspective which suggests that a person's thoughts and behaviour can be explained by physical malfunctioning, usually of neurotransmitters within the brain. Since it is clear that social and environmental factors have an impact on physical processes, an organic approach does not discount these influences, but views physical malfunctioning as the underlying cause of problems. Therefore primary emphasis is placed on physical interventions – usually drugs – to alleviate problems. It is worth noting that an 'illness'/'cure' model is not confined to doctors or psychiatrists but widely held by a range of clinicians and those outside mental health services. At the same time, there have been a number of doctors who have been vocal in their opposition to an organic perspective (c.f. Laing 1960, Szasz 1961, Romme et al 1992, Thomas 1997).

A 'pure' organic model is probably adopted by few clinicians; differences between exponents of different perspectives typically revolve around the extent of biological determinism and the efficacy of pharmacological and non-pharmacological interventions. Most clinicians would accept that the social and physical environment play a contributing role in the development of a person's difficulties, and would adopt some form of 'stress-vulnerability' perspective (Falloon et al 1984, Tarrier 1992, Brooker et al 1994). This approach maintains that people are more or less vulnerable (as a result of their experiences or biology) to the social stressors that might precipitate mental health problems.

Opposition to the organic model has been extensive from both clinicians (c.f. Boyle 1993, Podvoll 1990, Barker 1999, Clarke 1999) and service-users (c.f. Chamberlin 1977, Read & Reynolds 1996, Barker et al 1999, Faulkner & Layzell 2000). We will not rehearse these arguments here. We would advocate a perspective which avoids prescribing the 'true' nature of mental distress/disability and accords the choice of model to the person whose experiences are being explained. A desire to promote choice of treatment and services must be accompanied by a similar choice in explanatory models.

Different models of madness derive from different constructions of the world and events within it, but none is 'true' in any absolute sense. There is nothing 'truer' about assorted neurotransmitters than there is about intrapsychic processes, inner children or various deities. (Perkins 1999)

Different understandings of mental health problems determine the way in which people view their difficulties and the type of help they seek (Perkins & Repper, 1998), but different models have important political and social implications.

In favour of the illness model, it has been argued that, by promoting the genetic and biochemical origins of 'madness', the associated discrimination and exclusion can be reduced (National Alliance of the Mentally Ill 1996). Such arguments assert that if the public comes to see mental illness as an illness like any other then the individuals affected will not be blamed for their problems, and discrimination will be diminished. Research indicates that the more responsible a person is considered to be for their difficulties the more discrimination they experience (Stangor & Crandor 2000). Therefore, if 'madness' is seen as an illness rather than as a moral weakness, then people will not be blamed for what they do because they cannot be responsible for their actions.

Such a perspective is often attractive to the families of people who experience mental health problems, as they often feel blamed for causing or maintaining their relatives' difficulties (Hatfield 1987). A biological model can absolve them of the guilt that they would otherwise feel for the difficulties of their kinfolk. Some service-users also find relief in a diagnosis of 'mental illness':

> ... it made sense of all the symptoms, but I hadn't thought of it myself ... It just made sense of not sleeping, waking up early and not being able to get to sleep and not being able to eat, being constantly worried about what was going to happen, that sort of thing. (cited in Faulkner & Layzell 2000)

> It is impossible for any sane person even to begin to imagine how I felt. It is also obvious to anyone with a shred of common sense that I was ill. Any characterisation of my behaviour as merely 'bizarre', that such an 'illness' attribution would then be an act of social control (to empower the medical profession), is clearly utterly absurd. (Chadwick 1997b).

> ... I found it kind of liberating. For a while I could receive the absolution I needed for failing to do the things I usually did. My relationships with friends and family improved: I had not simply become lazy, unreliable and extremely irritable, now there was something 'wrong'. (Perkins 1999)

It is the popular assumption that 'illness' is a time-limited phenomenon. You get ill, you call in sick to your work, cancel social engagements, take to your bed, imbibe appropriate medicaments, and get better. This may be entirely appropriate during circumscribed crises. If there are time-limited periods when mental health problems preclude you from meeting all your work and social obligations, it is useful to be relieved of these responsibilities until you get back on an even keel and can resume them.

However, problems arise because the idea of 'mental illness' is used to refer not only to time-limited crises, but to ongoing problems. Even if the 'illlness' goes away, the label of 'mental illness' often does not. And when the 'illness' continues, roles and responsibilities are suspended indefinitely and it is all too easy to become nothing but your 'illness':

> *To live 18 years with a diagnosed illness is no incentive for a positive self-image. Illness is a one-way street, especially when experts toss the concept of cure out of the window and congratulate themselves on candour. The idea of illness that can never go away is not a dynamic, liberating force. Illness creates victims. While we harbour thoughts of emotional distress as some kind of deadly plague, it is not unrealistic to expect that many so-called victims will lead limited, powerless and unfulfilling lives.* (Campbell 1996a)

An illness perspective may be positive and optimistic if a 'cure' is possible and rapid, but this is often not the case in relation to mental health problems. 'Cures' are far from sure and, even if symptoms can be completely alleviated, discrimination often continues on the basis of the person's history of mental illness.

There are a number reasons why an 'illness like any other' model fails to reduce discrimination and exclusion in the mental health arena (Sayce 2000). First, it all too easily replaces hatred and blame with pity and patronising attitudes: 'The poor things, they cannot help it.' To be the object of pity is not a powerful or valued role. Second, irreversible genetic explanations of 'mental illness' have resulted in some of the worst types of abusive discrimination and extreme exclusion, exemplified by the eugenics movement of the 1930s, and its elimination of 'useless eaters' (Birley 1999). Third, if 'mental illness' were seen like influenza or measles then perhaps the idea of 'illness' would reduce discrimination. However, in the physical domain, there is no evidence that an 'illness' construction reduces discrimination. The organic basis of physical and sensory impairments is uncontested, yet discrimination and exclusion remain rife. It was an illness – polio – that left Franklin Delano Roosevelt paralysed from the waist down, yet in the 1920s and 1930s he had to hide his impairments in order to be acceptable as President. Gallagher (1999) described his intense efforts 'to minimise the extent of his handicap, to make it unnoticed when possible and palatable when it was noticed ... This was FDR's splendid deception.' Finally, in removing blame, an 'illness' approach also removes responsibility. Behaviour is seen as a consequence of illness ('they cannot help it') and therefore rights and citizenship are denied.

> *Unlike physical illnesses, which affect particular parts of the body, mental illnesses affect that abstraction known as the mind. Once it has been decided that a person has a sick mind, enormous social consequences ensue. A finding of mental illness, which is often a judicial, as well as a*

medical, determination frequently results in loss of liberty. People labelled mentally ill are usually presumed to be incapable of exercising decision-making power in their own best interests ... People who are labelled mentally ill become part of a system that deprives them of control over their life as part of their treatment. (Chamberlin 1977)

And if this 'treatment' is less than wholly successful, the loss of rights and control becomes a permanent state of affairs.

In the physical arena, few would see as 'ill' someone who is in a wheelchair, blind, or deaf: they would be seen as disabled. And the action considered appropriate in relation to disability is quite different from that appropriate in the context of illness. In the face of temporary illness it may be useful to suspend roles and responsibilities – to put life on 'hold' until the problems diminish – but this would be wholly inappropriate in the context of disability. Disability is something with which you must live your life; if you put your life on hold then it will be 'on hold' for ever.

With disability comes rights. There is now legislation which offers some protection against discrimination on the grounds of disability in a number of countries from the USA to China. In Britain, the 1995 Disability Discrimination Act specifically includes people who experience mental health problems and learning difficulties. Such legislation, together with the changes which it demands, and the campaigning which surrounds it, offer probably the most promising avenue for fighting discrimination and combating exclusion, through cross-disability alliances:

User/survivors and other disabled people all share discrimination on the basis of some presumed 'imperfection' of body, mind or emotion and can join together in challenging the very idea of perfection. Together they can tackle the common experience of massive exclusion ... (Sayce 2000)

Almost all the problems that persons with physical disabilities face are shared by persons with psychiatric disabilities (for example difficulty in accessing housing, employment, and community services) ... we have grown closer to the disability community and discovered the commonalities that we share. (Chamberlin 1993)

It is our contention that there is much to be gained at social/political and individual levels from a social disability model for mental health problems. Cognitive and emotional problems, like mobility and sensory impairments, are not disabling in and of themselves; it is the associated discrimination and exclusion that are disabling.

The social model of disability holds that a person is disabled if he or she is, for example, blind, and experiences barriers and exclusion as a result.

The term is not limited to those who 'use' blindness services nor to people who are 'surviving'. It covers everyone affected by discrimination on the grounds of the supposed imperfection of disability. It allows for transforming negative associations into positive ones, through disability pride. (Sayce 2000)

A disability perspective does not presuppose any particular construction of mental health problems. It can accommodate people who believe that their difficulties are organic, social, psychological, or spiritual in nature, as well as those who see their problems as a consequence of traumatic abuse or devastating events. A social model of disability can also accommodate people who no longer have any cognitive or emotional problems, but who continue to experience discrimination because of their history of such difficulties, and those who believe that their problems arise only from the damage wrought on them by an oppressive mental health system.

A social disability model entails a change in thinking, i.e. a change in focus from symptoms and cures to people's lives outwith their illness. When we think about disability, we think about inclusion: access to roles, activities and facilities. We think about people's interests, aspirations and achievements. Whereas an 'illness' perspective focuses on changing people (making them 'fit in' by decreasing their symptoms), within a social model of disability, changing the world becomes the primary consideration. It prioritises enabling people to do the things they want to do and to live the lives they wish to live (with the adaptations, supports and aids, as well as the social and policy changes, that they need in order to do so). Such a shift in vision can already be seen in relation to psychiatric rehabilitation (c.f. Bennett 1978) but could usefully be extended throughout the mental health services.

Mental health problems are not a full time job – we have lives to lead. Any services, or treatments, or interventions, or supports must be judged in these terms – how much they allow us to lead the lives we wish to lead. (Perkins 2000)

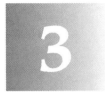

The realities of social exclusion

INTRODUCTION

You become a no-thing in a no-world and you are not. (Unziker 1989)

The exclusion of people defined as mad from their communities and society in general is nothing new. Although 'community care' may have ended incarceration in remote asylums, rejection and exclusion are as much a reality of life for people with mental health problems as they have ever been. Indeed, those diagnosed with a significant mental illness are amongst the most excluded in society (Sayce & Measey 1999, Sayce & Morris 1999, Sayce 2000, 2001b).

There is mounting evidence of the discrimination experienced by people with mental health problems in Britain. This discrimination results in their systematic exclusion from society. Social exclusion operates in all areas of life – daily living, work and training, and access to services... (Dunn 1999)

As Dahrendorf (1985) suggests, 'many in the majority class wish they would simply go away' – a sentiment reflected in the slogan 'Schizophrenics Go Home' daubed on a van outside a new residential facility for people with mental health problems (Repper et al 1997). The extent of this exclusion was revealed in a survey of 778 people with mental health problems (Read & Baker 1996):

- ◆ 34% had been dismissed or forced to resign from jobs
- ◆ 69% had been put off applying for jobs for fear of unfair treatment
- ◆ 47% had been abused or harassed in public (11% had been physically attacked)
- ◆ 26% had been forced to move home because of harassment

◆ 50% felt they had been unfairly treated by physical health services
◆ 33% complained that their GP had treated them unfairly
◆ 25% had been turned down by insurance or finance companies.

The consequences of such social exclusion are enormous. Unemployment alone, with its associated poverty, social isolation and loss of status, significantly increases disability and impedes recovery. It is increasingly recognised that discrimination and exclusion are at least as disabling as the problems that led to the diagnosis of mental health problems in the first place (Wing & Brown 1970, Deegan 1988, Rogers 1995, Perkins & Repper 1996, Sartorius 2000) .

For many years, madness has been a taboo subject, hidden away, not discussed (Repper 2000b). For the vast majority of the population, negative media images are the primary source of information about mental health problems. Philo et al (1993) have shown that such imagery overrides evidence gained from personal experience. Negative portrayals of mental health problems typically take two forms. On the one hand, people with mental health problems are seen as incompetent, i.e. unable to participate fully in society and in need of others to look after them and make decisions for them. As Chadwick (1997b) writes: 'You are bound to come across people who think your mental disorder disqualifies you a priori from having *anything* useful or meaningful to say about anything.' The views of those who experience mental distress and disability are seen as, by definition, invalid:

In the media, this is conveyed by the chronic absence of users' voices – everyone else from clinician to relative, seeming more 'worth listening to' – and by articles commenting on the self-evident absurdity of 'patients running the asylum'. A rash of such stories appeared in Britain in the 1990s criticising Patients Councils . . . (Sayce 2000)

The achievements of those who have mental health problems are rarely covered.

On the other hand, the media present an alarming picture of 'a rising tide of killings' by 'mad axe murderers'. Philo et al (1993) found that two-thirds of media coverage of mental health issues is negative and alarmist – a trend that is on the increase.

The media make people afraid of us. One person is violent and it's all over the press and then people think it applies to everyone who's been in hospital. If you're a big man like me it's worse. People cross the street to avoid me. (cited in Rose 1996)

The media association between madness, community care and violence, and the popular panic that ensues, fly in the face of evidence. Taylor & Gunn

(1999) reviewed Home Office criminal statistics for England and Wales between 1967 and 1995 (the period of major closure of mental hospitals and the development of community care). They found that the proportion of homicides committed by people with a mental disorder *fell* from 35 to 11.5%. As Sayce (2000) points out:

> *Factors more predictive [of violence] than mental illness – being young and male and the use of alcohol or drugs – receive less fearful media attention than 'psycho-killer' stories and there are no campaigns calling for the preventive detention of men who drink and assault their partners equivalent to those demanding the detention of mental patients.*

When elected in 1997, the UK Labour Government expressed concern about the social exclusion of many disadvantaged groups and declared an intention to reduce this exclusion. A 'Social Exclusion Unit' was formed which defined social exclusion as 'a shorthand for what can happen when individuals or areas suffer from a combination of linked problems such as unemployment, poor skills, low incomes, poor housing, high crime environments, bad health and family breakdown.' (Social Exclusion Unit 1999). Exclusion, however, amounts to more than either the causes or the effects of economic disadvantage. Duffy (1995) refers to 'a broader concept than poverty, encompassing not only low material means, but the inability to participate effectively in economic, social, political and cultural life, and in some characterisations, alienation and distance from mainstream society.' More specifically, in relation to people with mental health problems, Sayce (2000) defines social exclusion as:

> *...the inter-locking and mutually compounding problems of impairment, discrimination, diminished social role, lack of economic and social participation and disability. Among the factors at play are lack of status, joblessness, lack of opportunities to establish a family, small or non-existent social networks, compounding race and other discriminations, repeated rejection and consequent restriction of hope and expectation.*

The relationship between mental health problems and social exclusion is complex. Many of the elements of exclusion, such as low income, unemployment and lack of social networks, are both the causes of such problems and a consequence of them. For example, unemployment leads to an increase in the risk of experiencing mental health problems (Smith 1985, Warr 1987). Yet pervasive employment discrimination ensures that the experience of mental health problems is also a cause of unemployment. The 2000 Labour Force Survey revealed that unemployment amongst those with mental health problems is alarmingly high, at 84% (Office of National Statistics, 2000) – far higher than that among people with sensory and physical impairments (Burchardt 2000).

The Mind Enquiry into social exclusion of people with mental health problems (Dunn 1999) outlines a number of factors that are both a consequence of mental health problems and interact with them to promote social exclusion. These factors are outlined below.

◆ Media stereotyping
◆ discrimination at work
◆ lack of access to educational and training opportunities
◆ unemployment
◆ poor income
◆ homelessness and poor housing
◆ lack of informal job contacts
◆ contact with the criminal justice system
◆ ostracisation by the wider community
◆ disrupted family and social networks
◆ adverse effects of prescribed drug treatments
◆ drug misuse
◆ physical health problems
◆ stigmatising health and social services.

The evidence presented at the Mind Enquiry '... was powerful testament to the "holistic" nature of social exclusion – both cause and effect are multifaceted and interconnected ... so that a simple cause and effect model cannot be applied.' (Dunn 1999).

THE REALITY OF DISCRIMINATION

Feeling different and being ostracised are everyday realities for people with mental health problems. Such experiences cut across all facets of life.

Daily Living

Sometimes the discrimination and exclusion experienced in the ordinary round of everyday life are quite subtle:

There's a whole minor set of things I had never really thought about until I experienced my own mental health problems. Things like the sidelong looks you get from pharmacists when you go along with a prescription for psychotropic medication. (cited in Dunn 1999)

People are uneasy and suspicious.

They're a bit stand-offish with me.

I talk to the people at the bus stop but they ignore me, they talk to each other but they reject me. (cited in Rose 1996)

Friends, family, people you meet everyday – people treat you differently.
Like they are treading on eggshells … they think that if they say the wrong
thing you're going to flare up or whatever. (cited in Repper et al 1998)

At other times, rejection takes more frightening forms. Read & Baker's
(1996) survey revealed people who had been attacked, had eggs thrown at
them, or who had had dog faeces put through their door, simply because they
were known to have mental health problems. As one 71-year-old man
recounted 'Various gangs in the district call me "nutter" and spit at me. The
gangs on the estate know I was a psychiatric patient and so I'm teased and
harassed.' (Read & Baker 1996).

As a result of such experiences, many people keep very quiet about their
mental health problems: 'I'd never tell them I've been in hospital, they wouldn't
talk to me.' (cited in Rose 1996). However, along with such silence comes a fear
of being 'found out':

A man from the local mental hospital came into the shop and everyone
talked about him once he'd gone. They said he shouldn't be allowed
out… I felt so embarrassed and worried they'd find out about me.

I don't tell people in the neighbourhood that I've been in hospital. The
pharmacist knows, though, because of my prescriptions. I worry that he'll
tell people. (cited in Rose 1996)

Day-to-day rejection and avoidance leads to a diminution of social networks:

Friends avoided me and would not let their children play with my chil-
dren any more. (cited in Read and Baker 1996)

I feel alone on the estate – they know about me and they shut me out.
(cited in Rose 1996)

When I went into psychiatric hospital the Minister didn't come to visit
me. He always visits people when they are in hospital. But he didn't visit
me. (cited in Sayce 2000)

Former friends and social contacts drift away, too often leaving the person
isolated and alone in their distress.

Service-user experiences of rejection in day-to-day life are echoed in the
reports of service providers. Repper et al (1997) found that over two-thirds of
the statutory and voluntary sector mental health providers she surveyed had
experienced 'nimby' ('not in my back yard') campaigns in response to proposed
community facilities for people with mental health problems. The main reasons for opposition from local residents were 'fear' – of violence, of threats to
children, and of effects on the neighbourhood. Given such perceptions of mental health service-users, it is not surprising that social networks become

'truncated' (Mueller 1980). In a study of 310 people with mental health problems, Holmes-Eber & Riger (1990) found that lengthy and repeated admissions were associated with smaller social networks. A survey of people with ongoing mental health problems revealed that 40% of those living in the community had no social contacts outside mental health services (Ford et al 1994).

The rejection and lack of social support resulting is disabling in and of itself; but it can also exacerbate mental health problems. Gourash (1978) has described four ways in which social support can prevent mental health problems: buffering the effects of stress; providing immediate and appropriate assistance; acting as a screening mechanism for people to identify when they need to ask for professional help; and to convey attitudes, values and norms that guide behaviour. Friends can help a person overcome feelings of helplessness and raise their self-esteem (Schradle and Dougher 1985), and social isolation has been associated with depression (Brown and Harris 1978), a deterioration in social skills (Birchwood 1992), and more extreme reactions to stressful life events (Cohen and Willis 1985). Social isolation is also exacerbated by unemployment.

Employment

This is my workplace. This is where I earn my definition, the place that tells me what I am. (Galloway 1991)

Employment is central to social inclusion and to the lives of most people. Bennett (1978) has described work (in contrast to occupational therapy) as the performance of tasks, within prescribed limits, to achieve goals set by others, who judge and reward you, *thereby linking the individual to society.* Work is more than just a source of income, since it provides social contact and social support, social status and identity, a means of structuring and occupying time, activity and involvement, and a sense of personal achievement (Jahoda et al 1933, Shepherd 1984, Rowland & Perkins 1988, Shepherd 1989, Nehring et al 1993, Pozner et al 1996).

For people who are already excluded because of their mental health problems, work takes on an even greater importance. People with such problems are particularly sensitive to the isolation and loss of structure, purpose, and identity that unemployment brings.

It boosts self-esteem and provides a sense of purpose and accomplishment. Work enables people to enter, or re-enter, the mainstream after psychiatric hospitalisation. (Rogers 1995)

Most people with mental health problems attach a high priority to work, but discrimination combined with lack of support and encouragement conspire to ensure that it is exceptionally hard for them.

I had a cleaning job for three years, but when I mentioned an appointment with a psychiatrist I received a letter the next week to say my services were no longer required. (Read & Baker 1996)

I was employed as a social worker, but after six months I went into hospital with depression ... my contract of employment was terminated despite reports provided by my GP and psychiatrist which stated that my illness didn't affect my work and they were prepared to sign me fit to return to work. (Read & Baker 1996)

Last year I was offered a position as a graduate programmer and I was pleased with the prospect of working in industry using the skills and knowledge I had gathered from my time at university. I was devastated to be told a week later that the offer had been withdrawn because my security clearance was not accepted due to me suffering a mental illness ... My details are now stored in a database that thousands of companies use, so my chances of gaining employment with other companies are non-existent. (Read & Baker 1996)

Even those people in work continue to experience discrimination. In a survey of 556 people conducted by The Mental Health Foundation (Bird 2001) the main problems reported by those in work included the following:

◆ lack of confidence
◆ feelings of stress and anxiety
◆ feelings of isolation and exclusion resulting in poor performance
◆ fear of disclosing mental health problems
◆ lack of understanding from others leading to stigma and discrimination and in some cases bullying
◆ feeling unable to cope with the social aspects of the work situation
◆ problems communicating
◆ being given demeaning jobs with few or no prospects.

Of the respondents not in work, 95% said that their mental health problems had affected their work prospects, most of the difficulties being due to lack of understanding (leading to stigma and discrimination), gaps in employment history (which are difficult to explain), problems completing medical questionnaires, fear of the reoccurrence of mental health problems, and the need for support and training in order to do the job.

The experiences of service-users are reflected in surveys of employers, which reveal a reluctance to consider employing people with a history of mental health problems (c.f. Manning & White 1995). Data collected by the Department of Work and Pensions (2001) show that, despite acute labour shortages, employers seeking to tap new labour pools continue to be reluctant to employ those who have experienced mental health problems: 62% were prepared to consider employing those with physical impairments, while only 37% said they would consider those with mental health difficulties. Glozier (1998) conducted a survey in which 200 personnel officers were sent vignettes of two potential employees. These vignettes were identical except that one person was said to have a diagnosis of depression and the other a diagnosis of diabetes. Predictably, the applicant with depression was far less likely to be considered for employment than the one with diabetes.

Negative stereotyping and discrimination is not, however, limited to employers: many mental health workers assume that people with mental health problems are unlikely to be able to work (Rinaldi 2000).

> *I'd love to go back to work ... earning your own money, being your own person ... but they won't let me back ... the GP and the doctors at the hospital say 'no'.* (cited in Repper et al 1998)

> *In 1971, I was 19 and had the same abilities and ambitions as any other 19-year-old. I hoped to make a place in the world for myself. But instead I was a patient in a state hospital ... One day I was summoned to the office of the vocational rehabilitation counselor ... he looked up and said 'Well, there's nothing much I have to offer you; I can see from your chart that you'll never be capable of holding a job.' Tears came to my eyes; I thought all the facts were in. At the age of 19, when most people are eagerly anticipating and planning for the future, I had been told that I had nothing to look forward to but a 'career' as a ward of the state.* (Rogers 1995)

In fact, this man has enjoyed a successful career and now occupies a very senior position.

Often mental health workers justify pessimism about service-user's ability to work on the grounds of 'being realistic'. However, it is important to note that such 'realism' is not consistent with the evidence (Secker & Membury 2000, Secker et al 2001). This shows that employment success is <u>not</u> related to diagnosis or severity of symptomatology (Anthony 1994, Anthony et al 1995); the services and supports available are the most important factor. Research indicates that, with appropriate assistance (often from mental health workers), at least 50% of those who experience serious ongoing mental health problems can gain and sustain employment (Bond et al 1997, 2001, Crowther et al 2001).

Employment discrimination often means that people are put off from applying for jobs – they simply give up. ['I must have written off for 20 or 30 jobs ... I got one reply.' (cited in Perkins et al 2000)]. Alternatively, discrimination can lead to many people choosing to keep their mental health problems hidden for fear of losing, or failing to get, jobs.

I always lied, no-one ever knew. On the health forms I always ticked 'No' in the box that says 'Have you ever had mental health problems?' (cited in Perkins et al 2000)

I was working in a solicitor's as a trainee receptionist. I couldn't tell my boss I had to see a psychiatrist every week, so I told him I was on a training scheme one day a week. (cited in Dunn 1999)

Indeed, it may be preferable to have been in prison than to have mental health problems as far as employment is concerned:

On two occasions I lied when I applied for jobs. On both these occasions I said that my two and a half year absence from employment was due to a term spent in prison. I was accepted for the first and short listed for the second. Whenever I have been truthful about my psychiatric past I have never been accepted for a job. (cited in Dunn 1999)

A criminal record can be 'spent' in many jobs under 'rehabilitation of offenders' legislation, but a psychiatric history should always be declared.

Maintaining silence can have negative effects. First, it means that people may be reluctant to seek help from psychiatric services or feel unable to ask for the assistance they need in order to sustain employment. It is unlikely that the excuse of a training scheme (see above) could be sustained indefinitely! Second, if the person's mental health problems do come to light then they can be dismissed for lying. Yet to tell the truth all too often has the same result, the choice being between the devil or the 'deep-blue sea'.

Although some employers have made efforts to change the situation (see, for example, Perkins 1998, Perkins et al 2000, and the work of some members of the Employers' Forum on Disability), unemployment remains the norm for those with mental health problems. And the consequences of unemployment – poverty, limited social networks, poor physical and mental health (Brenner 1979, Smith 1985) – are all factors implicated in social exclusion (Social Exclusion Unit 1999). Thus, not only is unemployment excluding in and of itself, but it leads to a range of other problems that aggravate this exclusion.

Living on a low income

Unemployment is typically linked with poverty or low income, which themselves reduce opportunities for a good quality of life. Bird (2001) identified two interlocking effects of having mental health problems and living on a low income. First, people were not able to afford items that many of us consider basic necessities: decent food and clothing, fuel bills, holidays, and social activities:

Because of my low income ... I go for foods with cheaper prices and those with special offers, I have not bought new clothes for years and have not been out for a meal, cinema or a holiday for more than 10 years.

Due to medication I have put on a lot of weight and I have outgrown my clothes but due to my income I cannot afford to buy new ones. (cited in Bird 2001)

Second, the effects of continually struggling to afford necessities and being unable to go out, buy presents, dress up and so on, affected people's self esteem, leading them to feel despondent and degraded.

Out of the blue your job has gone, with it any financial security you may have had. At a stroke, you have no purpose in life, and no contact with other people. You find yourself totally isolated from the rest of the world. No one telephones you. Much less writes. No one seems to care if you're alive or dead.

All in all I find the experience of being on a low income degrading. I feel I am being punished for being ill and as if it is my fault which in turn makes me more depressed. You see others buying such lovely things and I can have none of it. It really hurts. (cited in Bird 2001)

FAMILY LIFE AND PARENTING

It has been estimated that between 40 and 60% of people with a diagnosis of schizophrenia live with their families (Fadden et al 1987, Kuipers 1993). Undoubtedly, these families provide an enormous amount of support and social contact: 'My mother really understands me.'; 'My brother helps me at work.' (cited in Rose 1996).

However, people have also reported that their mental health problems have resulted in exclusion from family life.

My in-laws wouldn't have me in the house for 10 years after my mental illness. My wife and daughter visited them, but I was not permitted. (cited in Sayce 2000)

My father won't give me a key to my own front door.
They want me to stay away.
My mother thinks I should be locked up. (cited in Rose 1996)

However, as Sayce (1997, 2000) describes, the greatest area of discrimination in family life occurs in relation to parenting. In their 1996 survey, Read & Baker found that 48% of women and 26% of men with mental health problems felt that their parenting abilities had been unfairly questioned. Once again, it is the negative stereotyping on the part of many mental health professionals about which many service-users complain. It is not uncommon for professionals to advise some people not to have children:

> *My consultant psychiatrist told my husband and I not to have children – 'they will be taken away, no doubt about it'. We now have a beautiful two and a half year old daughter; we are, to quote our GP, 'excellent parents' and our care of our daughter is 'always of a high standard'.* (cited in Read & Baker 1996)

> *My ex-husband's got them and won't let me see them. The courts gave him custody because I've been in hospital. I want to see them so much.* (cited in Rose 1996)

Perkins (1992) has described the devastating impact – including suicide – wrought on the lives of women with mental health problems who have had their children taken into care. Yet, where specific attempts have been made to provide support to parents with mental health problems, things can be different. For example, the Chicago Mother's Project (Zeitz 1995) provides intensive outreach support and a day-programme for mothers with such difficulties who would otherwise have had their children removed by the courts. This assistance has enabled many mothers and their children to stay together. Hardman (1997) challenges popular assumptions that such continued contact has a detrimental effect on the children. Herself the daughter of a mother with severe and enduring mental health problems, she has described the negative impact of having been separated from her mother. She was denied all contact, until she was an adult and able to decide for herself to resume contact.

Although the majority of children born to a parent with schizophrenia do not develop the illness, and of 89% of people who do develop schizophrenia, neither of their parents is affected (McGuffin et al 1995, Darton 1998), advice against parenting may also be given in the form of 'genetic counselling':

> *To cite but one possible future application [of genetic research into schizophrenia], mental health nurses may well be involved in the genetic counselling of families of those with schizophrenia and other mental disorders'.* (Gournay 1996)

The assumption of such 'genetic counselling' is that life with a mental health problem is 'not worth living' and that people should avoid having children who might be saddled with the 'burden'. This, of course, implies that the life of the parent who already has mental health problems must be worthless. What could be more devaluing than a mental health professional implying that it would be better if you hadn't been born? As the highly successful researcher and Professor of Psychiatry, Kay Jamison, who also has a diagnosis of manic depression, remembers:

In an icy and imperious voice that – I can hear to this day he [the doctor] stated – as though it were God's truth, which no doubt he felt it was – 'You shouldn't have children. You have manic depressive illness'. I felt sick, unbelievably and utterly sick, and deeply humiliated. Determined to resist being provoked into what would, without question, be interpreted as irrational behaviour, I asked him if his concerns about my having children stemmed from the fact that, because of my illness, he thought I would be an inadequate mother or simply that he thought it best to avoid bringing another manic- depressive into the world. Ignoring or missing my sarcasm, he replied 'both'.... I walked across the street to my car, sat down, shaking, and sobbed until I was exhausted. (Jamison 1995a)

ACCESS TO SERVICES AND ACTIVITIES

We would not wish to imply that everyone is excluded by all, or even the majority, of agencies. However, the experience of discrimination in all areas of life remains a day-to-day reality. Widespread negative attitudes resulting in discrimination have touched all areas of society including the police, housing and benefits agencies, businesses, insurance companies, community organisations, churches, clubs, physical health services, and mental health services themselves.

This man was sexually harassing me and I went to the police station for help. I said I wanted to take out an injunction. They said I couldn't because I was a mental patient. I don't think it's right. (cited in Rose 1996)

When I fill in an insurance form I have to put down about my depression. I got refusals from three companies I tried. (cited in Dunn 1999)

I moved house when I was eight months pregnant, and my midwife wrote 'hypomanic' in large red letters across my notes. No GP in my new area would take me on. (cited in Read & Baker 1996)

I've changed my church because at the last one they were terrible about mentally ill people. (cited in Rose 1996)

A young man ... had been going tramping [hiking] for some time with this club and really enjoyed it. One day he finally felt comfortable enough with his fellow trampers to state that he suffered from schizophrenia but that it was well managed. A week later his parents received a call from the tramping club to say that they would prefer that he did not attend. (Peters 1997, cited in Sayce 2000)

And then there's the problem with never being allowed to get a headache: if you take a prescription for antidepressants to a chemist, they will not let you simultaneously buy paracetamol or aspirin. (cited in Dunn 1999)

They [The Benefits Agency] treat you as a mental case. They see people before me because they think it doesn't matter if someone like me has to wait. (cited in Rose 1996)

When you want to organise a mortgage and get life cover, all the medical history that is in the GP's notes is sent to the insurance company. They say 'Oh this guy's been in hospital, on lithium, all these other drugs, let's put a loading on.' I've got a 60 per cent loading on my insurance cover. (cited in Dunn 1999)

They [the housing provider] think they can come into my flat without permission. (cited in Rose 1996)

They treat you like a child or worse. (cited in Rose 1996)

Every genuine illness I have had over the last twenty years has been dismissed as anxiety, depression or stress. (cited in Read & Baker 1996)

This tendency to dismiss complaints of physical health problems as a product of mental health difficulties is worrying. The National Psychiatric Morbidity Survey (see Harris & Barraclough 1998) showed higher levels of physical ill-health and higher rates of death among those with mental health problems compared with the rest of the population, and those with more serious mental health difficulties often have undiagnosed/untreated physical health problems (c.f. Harris & Barraclough 1998, Allebeck 1989).

AWAY FROM THE SHADOW OF THE PAST

The discrimination against people with mental health problems which gives rise to social exclusion starts from the identification of difference. But difference alone does not lead to discrimination: it is the way that difference is valued that is the key. World-class athletes and geniuses are 'different', but this difference is celebrated. The celebration of those differences that have been labelled 'madness' is rare; instead, they are viewed as 'imperfections' and those with them are seen as a threat to social order.

Inclusion cannot be contingent upon 'perfection' or 'sameness', however, for this is the road to the horrors of the eugenics movement, the compulsory sterilisation movement, and the Nazi euthanasia programmes. Compulsory sterilisation in the USA began in 1907, and some 60 000 people were sterilised, often without being informed about what was being done to them. Many European countries have seen similar programmes. From 1939 in Nazi Germany, at least 250 000 people with mental and physical impairments were considered to be 'useless eaters' – 'unworthy of life' – and therefore gassed, shot, or killed by lethal injection.

Records from the era show a meticulous calculation of the savings in potatoes, margarine, quark and jam for those people who had been 'disinfected' (killed). School mathematics books posed questions including: 'The construction of a lunatic asylum costs 6 million marks. How many houses at 15,000 marks each could have been built for that amount?' The lives of people with problems such as schizophrenia and manic depression had been declared to be not worth the expense. (Sayce 2000, based on information from the United States Holocaust Memorial Museum 1996)

Although such atrocities – such extreme forms of 'social exclusion' – are far removed from life in the 21st century, they are based on similar ideas about the worth of people who have mental health problems.

Many circumstances of Germany in the 1920s are not very different from our own. There is still discrimination (including the allocation of funds for services) against the mentally ill or handicapped, a preoccupation with the cost of care – particularly for old people. The question of euthanasia and assisted suicide for the incurably ill is very actively debated, as is the issue of 'the quality of life' (QALY). [Williams 1985.] Some of these approaches have a sinister ring. For instance the essence of QALY is that it takes one year of healthy life expectancy to be worth one, but regards a year of unhealthy life expectancy as worth less than one.... If being dead is worth zero, it is, in principle, possible for a QALY to be negative i.e. for the quality of someone's life to be judged as worse than being dead. (Birley 1999)

One might hope and assume that this appalling history is over. In fact, we are still living in the shadow of its ideas. (Sayce 2000)

When we forget that people with mental illness share a common humanity with us, then the human is stripped from the human services and the stage is set for the emergence of the inhuman and the inhumane. (Deegan 1990)

It is the diversity that exists within society that renders it strong, and it is the co-operation and contribution of people with diverse backgrounds and experiences – including those who experience mental health problems – that renders it supportive, flexible and tolerant.

Social exclusion is disabling in its own right, but when combined with the cognitive and emotional difficulties associated with mental health problems the impact is magnified. A vicious cycle is established which prevents people from developing and using their talents, which saps self-confidence, and which exacerbates their mental health difficulties, thus depriving society of the contribution that they could make. By contrast, Sayce (2000) describes social inclusion in the following terms:

a virtuous circle of improved rights of access to the social and economic world, new opportunities, recovery of status and meaning, and reduced impact of disability. Key issues will be availability of a range of opportunities that users can choose to pursue, with support or adjustments where necessary.

Mental health workers often talk about the discrimination and exclusion that exists in the wider community, but we must also attend to our own 'backyard'. Legal and policy changes are important, but so are changes in attitudes and practices within the mental health services. As mental health workers, we may not be able to change the world, but our values can influence the lives of individuals with whom we work – for good or ill.

As I look back over the history of services for people with mental illness I fail to see the common ground upon which both persons with mental illness and those who seek to serve them stand. Instead I see those who stand on higher ground and those who are left to stand or cower on lower ground. Service models and treatment theories come and go. But the relationship between those who have been diagnosed with mental illness and those who do not remains essentially unchanged. (Deegan 1989)

Sartorius (2000) has argued that stigma and discrimination are 'the major problems facing psychiatry today' and 'the most serious obstacle to progress in the field of psychiatry'. He exhorts mental health workers to look to their own practices and ideas and the way in which these perpetuate negative and devaluing attitudes, discrimination and exclusion.

4

The individual's recovery journey: towards a model for mental health practice

INTRODUCTION

In the mental health services we are used to thinking about people's experience in terms of the supports and interventions that mental health workers provide. We think in terms of in-patient facilities, outreach services, medication, occupational therapy, art therapy, and 'psychosocial interventions'. We think of symptom reduction and discharge as indices of success. This is the wrong place to start. Everyone who experiences mental health problems faces the challenge of recovery, i.e. rebuilding a meaningful and valued life. Whether a person's problems are time-limited or ongoing, whether or not their symptoms can be eliminated, they face the task of living with, and growing beyond, what has happened to them. The help offered by mental health workers needs to be considered in terms of the extent to which they facilitate, or hinder, this process of recovery.

If we are to facilitate recovery, then we must think about the challenges people face and the impact of what we do on a person's particular journey. An understanding of the process of recovery is essential to the development of effective treatment, support and rehabilitation (Farkas et al 1999). This can only be gained from the accounts of people who have themselves faced the challenge of recovery. Such accounts are widely available and essential reading for mental health workers. Stories of recovery are increasingly related at conferences, in academic journals, and in specific collections.

WHAT IS RECOVERY?

> Recovery refers to the lived or real life experience of people as they accept and overcome the challenge of the disability ... they experience themselves as recovering a new sense of self and of purpose within and beyond the limits of the disability. (Deegan 1988)

Unlike so many ideas in the mental health arena, the concept of recovery from mental health problems did not come from academics and professionals. Instead, it emerged from the writing of people who themselves face the challenge of life with mental health problems (e.g. Houghton 1982, Lovejoy 1982, Deegan 1988, 1993, 1996, 1999, Leete 1988a, 1989, Unziker 1989, McDermott 1990, Spaniol & Koehler 1994, Read & Reynolds 1996, Chadwick 1997b, Reeves 1998, May 2000). Drawing on these accounts, Anthony (1993) has described recovery as:

> *...a deeply personal, unique process of changing one's attitudes, values, feelings, goals, skills, and/or roles. It is a way of living a satisfying, hopeful, and contributing life even with limitations caused by illness. Recovery involves the development of new meaning and purpose in one's life as one grows beyond the catastrophic effects of mental illness.*

Experiencing serious mental health problems is a catastrophic and life-changing experience. There is no going back to how life was before the problems started. Those bridges are burnt. But it is not the end of life – there is a way forward. Recovery is possible.

◆ *Recovery is not the same as cure*. It does not mean that all suffering has disappeared, that all symptoms have been removed, or that functioning has been completely restored. Rather, remaining symptoms and problems interfere less with a person's life.

> *One of the biggest lessons I have had to accept is that recovery is not the same thing as being cured. After 21 years of living with this thing it still hasn't gone away.* (Deegan 1993)

◆ *Recovery is about growth.*

> *Recovery to me is not only coming to terms with what has happened in my own life, the dark side of me and the things I have done, but having grown as an individual because of my experiences. Focusing on this experience as a source of growth has been the source of inspiration for recovery. I can now look back in time and know that everything that happened... helped me to become the person I am today...* (Reeves 1998)

It is all too easy for a person to become nothing other than their 'illness': 'a schizophrenic', 'a manic depressive': 'Schizophrenia is an "I am" illness, one which may take over and redefine the identity of a person' (Estroff 1989). People with mental health problems are more than embodiments of their 'illness'. Recovery involves redefining identity in a way which includes, but moves beyond, that 'illness'. Recovery is important whether or not a person's symptoms can be cured. It involves overcoming not only the challenge of mental health difficulties themselves, but also the effects of the discrimination and exclusion which accompany them.

My recovery was about how to gain other people's confidence in my abilities and potential … in my own experience the toughest part was changing other people's expectations of what I could do. Combating a disempowering sense of being undervalued … (May 2000)

◆ *Recovery does not refer to an end-product or a result.* It is not an outcome but a continuing journey.

Recovery is a process, not an end point or destination. Recovery is an attitude, a way of approaching the day and the challenges I face … . I know I have certain limitations and things I can't do. But rather than letting these limitations be occasions for despair and giving up, I have learned that in knowing what I can't do, I also open up the possibilities of all I can do. (Deegan 1993)

◆ *Recovery can, and does, occur without professional intervention.* A person's own resources and those available to him/her outside the mental health system are central to the process. There are many paths to recovery, including choosing not to be involved with the mental health system (Anthony 1993). Recovery is not a professional intervention, like medication or therapy, and mental health workers do not hold the key. Many people have described the enormous support they have received from others who have faced a similar challenge (Chamberlin 1995, May 2000). The challenge faced by us as practitioners is to facilitate recovery, but we can also hinder it.

◆ *A recovery vision is not limited to a particular theory about the nature and causes of mental health problems.* Some writers (e.g. Chamberlin 1995, May 1999) have spoken eloquently about the disabling impact of the traditional 'organic' models. However, as Anthony (1993) points out, a recovery vision does not commit one to a social, a psychological, a spiritual, or an organic understanding of distress and disability, nor to the use or non-use of medical interventions. Whatever understanding of their situation a person comes to, recovery is an equally important process.

◆ *Recovery is not specific to people with mental health problems.* Everyone experiences the challenge of recovery at some point in life, e.g. when someone we love dies, or when we experience losses, traumas, illnesses, or injuries.

Recovery is a process of healing physically and emotionally, of adjusting one's attitudes, feelings, perceptions, beliefs, roles and goals in life. It is a painful process, yet often one of self-discovery, self-renewal and transformation. Recovery is a deeply emotional process. Recovery involves creating a new personal vision for one's self. (Spaniol et al 1997)

◆ *Recovery is about taking back control over one's life.* Mental health problems are often presented and perceived as uncontrollable, or their control is seen as the province of experts. Recovery involves a person taking back control.

> *Over the years I have learned different ways of helping myself. Sometimes I use medications, therapy, self-help and mutual support groups, friends, my relationship with God, work, exercise, spending time in nature – all of these measures help me remain whole and healthy, even though I have a disability.* (Deegan 1993)

◆ *Recovery is not a linear process.*

> *The recovery process is ... a series of small beginnings and very small steps. At times our course is erratic and we falter, slide back, re-group and start again ...* (Deegan 1988)

Relapse is not 'failure', but a part of the recovery process.

> *I have found that although my symptoms may seem ... worse, relapsing ... is not the same thing as 'having a breakdown'.... rather I am breaking out or breaking through ... out of some fear-filled place where I have been trapped ... through to new ways of trusting people and myself ... It means I am growing, breaking out of old fears and into new worlds – learning to make friends and keep them, to trust people, and to love people.* (Deegan 1993)

◆ Everyone's recovery journey is different and deeply personal. There are no rules of recovery, no formula for 'success'.

> *Everyone's journey of recovery is unique. Each of us must find our own way and no-one can do it for us.* (Deegan 1993)

> *Once recovery becomes systematised, you've got it wrong. Once it is reduced to a set of principles it is wrong. It is a unique and individualised process.* (Deegan 1999)

FROM WHAT ARE PEOPLE RECOVERING?

People who have been diagnosed with mental health problems are recovering from the multi-faceted catastrophe of that experience. This is likely to include the following:

◆ the multiple and often recurring traumas of the symptoms themselves
◆ the treatment of the illness, including the side-effects of medication and the stigma associated with contact with mental health services

◆ negative attitudes and prognoses of professionals ('You have a chronic illness.', 'You will not be able to work.' 'You'll always need help, drugs.', and so on)

◆ lack of appropriate skills in professionals (whose primary concern is typically the relief of symptoms) to help people to rebuild their lives

◆ devaluing and disempowering services which encourage passivity, where 'them and us' attitudes prevail, and where the physical environment is often depressing and inadequate

◆ lack of opportunities to engage in valued activities in line with interests and aspirations

◆ the many manifestations of discrimination and social exclusion.

Too often, mental health workers do not fully appreciate the range of traumas experienced by people with mental health problems. Professional training and practice – whether it be in medicine, nursing, social work, psychology, or occupational and other therapies – typically focus on the problems associated with the 'illness' itself. The impact of the other sources of trauma with which the person must grapple typically receive scant attention. As Spaniol et al (1997) showed, 'This has left many people with mental illness feeling devalued and ignored and has resulted in mistrust and alienation from the mental health system.' It is these multiple and interlocking traumas that have such a devastating impact on people's lives, often leaving them disconnected from themselves, from friends and family, from the communities in which they live, and from meaning and purpose in life. Unless mental health workers understand and address this complex range of barriers, we may inadvertently impede recovery by alienating people from the services that are supposed to assist them.

Spaniol et al (1997) describe four types of impact that the trauma associated with a diagnosis of mental health problems can have on an individual: loss of a sense of self; loss of power; loss of meaning; and loss of hope.

Loss of a sense of self

With time and experience, everyone develops a sense of who they are: this sense of self is profoundly challenged and fragmented by the experience of mental health problems (Estroff 1989). Within each person who has faced mental health problems there remains a persistent, healthy self trying to survive. But this is all too easily eclipsed by the identity of 'mental patient', which tends to mask all other identities. Often, mental health workers know little about people's lives prior to their illnesses, knowing them only during their 'mental patient' phase.

From a psychosocial perspective, chronicity involves the transformation of a prior, enduring, known and valued self into a devalued, passive and dysfunctional self (Estroff 1989, Davidson & Strauss 1992). This has a profoundly negative impact on the recovery process. A person's sense of self affects the whole range of their vocational, intellectual, social, emotional and spiritual functioning (Davidson & Strauss 1992). Recovery involves integrating what has happened to you into your former sense of self and developing a new, valued and valuable sense of identity. If no one understands and values the 'you' that is now masked by the identity of 'mental patient', then you become isolated and alienated from others.

Loss of Power

The experiences of diagnosis and using mental health services involve loss of agency, choice and the ability to determine your own interests. Symptoms can erode a person's sense of control, and this loss of confidence is compounded by services where the 'expert knows best' (Bockes 1989). The prevailing view that people with mental health problems are not able to determine what is best for themselves remains widespread. If no one else believes that you can help yourself, then it is difficult to see yourself as able to do so. Recovery is about active agency: retaining or taking back control over your life. Unless mental health workers can help people to take back control, we impede the recovery process.

Loss of meaning

Meaning in life is connected to the various roles that we adopt. Mental health problems all too often result in loss of valued roles as worker, wife, mother, football player, etc . . . . . People see their non-disabled peers doing the things that they had planned to do – going to college, getting married, pursuing their careers – while they are left behind. Often it is believed that such roles are beyond the reach of people with mental health problems. And if everyone tells you that you cannot do things, you have two choices. You can believe what they say and give up, or you can reject their bleak prognostications, further isolate yourself from former friends, family and mental health services, and keep trying. If, as mental health workers, we cannot be optimistic about the possibilities for meaningful and valued lives for people with mental health problems, then we impede the recovery process.

Loss of hope

The accumulation of traumatising and devaluing experiences that typically accompany mental health problems can lead a person to abandon hope. If a person can see no possibility of a positive future then it is all too easy to give up trying to do anything at all. Lovejoy (1982) emphasised that recovery is impossible without hope. It is hope that provides the courage to change, to trust others and to try things out. It is not surprising that high levels of 'hopelessness' when a person first experiences mental health problems are predictive of a poor outcome (Aguilar et al 1997). The challenge seems too great. People give up. Without hope, rebuilding your life is not possible. If mental health workers cannot foster hope, then they cannot assist in the recovery process. Hope is the key to recovery (Adams & Partree 1998).

WHAT MIGHT RECOVERY INVOLVE?

People must find their own individual paths for recovery and set about rebuilding their selves and futures in their own ways. A brief look at the writings of those who have faced this task is ample testimony to the personal, unique and very individual nature of their journeys. However, a number of authors have identified common features that may be involved in the recovery process (see, for example, Deegan 1988, 1993, 1996, Anthony 1993, Spaniol & Koehler 1994, Spaniol et al 1997, Vincent 1999, Young & Ensing 1999, May 2000). These must not be taken as a recipe or set of predetermined stages. We present them here in order to illustrate the areas of which mental health professionals must be aware in order to facilitate the recovery process. Although, for the purposes of description, each area is described separately, it will become clear that all are intimately interrelated.

Restoring Hope

The accounts of people who have experienced mental health problems consistently, and poignantly, emphasise the importance of hope – a perspective shared by many professionals (Marcel 1962, Kubler-Ross 1969, Stotland 1969, Brunner 1972, Dufault & Martocchio 1985, Plugge 1979, Farran et al 1995, Holdcraft & Williamson 1991). Lindsey (1976) describes hope as an 'anchor, stabilising our lives in the present and giving life meaning, direction and optimism'. It is 'neither passive waiting nor unrealistic forcing of circumstances that cannot occur, a state involving an inner readiness and activeness, a psychic concomitant to life and to psychosocial and spiritual growth' (Fromm 1968).

There exists a considerable body of research into the importance of hope in coping with physical illnesses (e.g. Hickey 1986). In the mental health arena, it has long been recognised that hope is one key to successful psychotherapy (Menninger 1959, Frank 1968). A number of studies have demonstrated a relationship between hopelessness and suicide (Drake & Cotton 1986, Beck et al 1990), and an increasing number of authors have stressed the importance of mental health workers' hopefulness in the treatment of schizophrenia and the process of rehabilitation (for example, Anthony et al 1990, Woodside et al 1994, Kirkpatrick et al 1995, Kanwal 1997).

But what is 'hope'?

A multidimensional dynamic life force characterised by a confident yet uncertain expectation of achieving a personally significant goal. (Dufault & Martocchio 1985)

Hope is a state characterised by an anticipation of a continued good state, an improved state, or a release from a perceived entrapment. The anticipation may or may not be founded on concrete, real world evidence. Hope is an anticipation of a future which is good and is based upon: mutuality (relationships with others), a sense of personal competence, coping ability, psychological well-being, purpose and meaning in life, as well as a sense of 'the possible'. (Miller 1992)

Such definitions emphasise the highly individual nature of hope. Hope relates to the achievement of goals that have a significance for the person concerned, and it does not have to relate to specific outcomes. Dufault & Martocchio (1985) distinguish between two major types of hope: (1) generalised hope related to a sense of some future beneficial developments but not linked to any particular concrete goal; (2) particularised hope related to a specific, valued outcome or state of being, like getting a job, getting married, or having a place of your own.

For people with mental health problems, hope lies at the heart of the individual's ability and willingness to take on the challenge of rebuilding and recovery. Acceptance of what has happened can be too terrifying in the absence of hope:

How can we accept the illness when we have no hope? Why should one pile despair on top of hopelessness? The combination could be fatal. So perhaps people are wise in not accepting the illness until they have the resources to deal with it. (Deegan 1996).

Hope counteracts depression and diminishes the risk of a person giving up: 'In the context of life threatening situations, hope functions as a life saving force for individuals who have been overwhelmed by despair.' (Russinova 1999). Hope motivates.

Deegan (1996) has drawn a distinction between optimism and hope. She characterises optimism as being like a cheer-leader – there for a brief period and then gone. Hope is a belief in one's self, a willingness to 'hang-in there', to persevere over the long haul that is involved in picking yourself up when you are knocked down. Hope is not a bolt of lightening; rather, it begins as a 'small and fragile flame' that can be either fanned or snuffed out.

It might be assumed that hope is related to the severity of a person's problems: the fewer the problems, the greater the hope. However, research conducted by Landeen et al (2000) shows that this is not the case. Among 100 people with a diagnosis of schizophrenia, they found no relationship between hope and symptom severity, nor was hope clearly related to financial factors, the number of social contacts, or the living situation. They found a strong relationship, however, between hope and quality of life. They concluded that material and clinical status are less important than the meaning that people attribute to their life situations. They argue that this points to the importance of discovering individual sources of meaning and value. Unfortunately, mental health services often fail to do this. Numerous people have described the way in which contact with such services and interactions with mental health workers have left them feeling discouraged and hopeless. Deegan (1990) has described this phenomenon as 'spirit breaking':

> *The experience of spirit breaking occurs as a result of those cumulative experiences in which we are humiliated and made to feel less than human, in which our will to live is deeply shaken or broken, in which our hopes are shattered and in which 'giving up', apathy and indifference become a way of surviving and protecting the last vestiges of the wounded self.*

Restoring hope – shedding the protection afforded by withdrawal, apathy and indifference – is a risky journey. It involves daring to trust people, risking disappointment, failure and further hurt. People may be reluctant to trust mental health workers and services which they believe have let them down in the past. People with a diagnosis of schizophrenia have identified four things that they see as important in 'igniting or nurturing their hope' (Kirkpatrick et al 2001).

Experiencing success

The experience of success had a number of dimensions, including finding a specific object of hope, setting realistic goals, accomplishing small daily tasks or changes, and achieving life goals in work. Vicarious experience may also be important. Hearing about the success of other people with the same diagnosis also served to inspire hope. A participant describing his feelings on hearing Bill McPhee, editor of the magazine *Schizophrenia Digest*, speaking about his ongoing struggle with schizophrenia (cited in Kirkpatrick et al 2001) was inspired: 'He had come from so far and was incapacitated for a number of years and to be functioning at that level gave me some feelings of hope.'

Taking control

In various ways, people had been able to understand, and gain control over, problems that had seemed uncontrollable: 'I have more control over my illness than I ever realised ... Knowing that gives me more hope because I know the next time when I start to get ill I can turn it around. You don't have to let your illness run your life.' (cited in Kirkpatrick et al 2001)

Finding meaning

In a variety of ways, people found value in their lives. This sometimes included religious and spiritual beliefs. A participant described '... feeling like there is some purpose in life. I'm not just a person here on earth meant to take, take, take, but I have something to give.' (cited in Kirkpatrick et al 2001)

Maintaining relationships

Aspects of relationships with friends, families and peers that were important in inspiring hope included being there, providing encouragement, showing understanding, and giving support: 'He listens to me and understands I am not well and that there are things I can and cannot do, but he always has the utmost faith in me.' (a participant describing his relationship with his brother; cited in Kirkpatrick et al 2001)

The Importance of Relationships

Relationships are central in fostering and maintaining hope (Byrne et al 1994). It is hard to sustain positive expectations for the future and a positive view of yourself when those around you offer only bleak prophecies. Hopeful support can be provided by relatives, friends, others who have experienced similar challenges, and mental health professionals:

> *The turning point in my life was ... where I started to get hope that I could actually make the leap from being sick to being well ...*
> *Dr. Charles believed I could. And Rev. Goodwin believed that I could ... Certain people believed that I could make the leap. And held that belief even when I didn't believe it myself.* (Donna, cited in Vincent 1999)

A common denominator of recovery is the presence of someone who 'stands by' you. This person is someone who believes in you when you find it hard to believe in yourself. It is very easy to lose sight of yourself as anything other than a mental patient when you enter psychiatric services, where all the attention is on your problems.

Professionals do not hold the key to recovery: relationships with others – friends, families, neighbours, colleagues – are more central. Although it can be important, there will always be limitations to the worker/client relationship because its very context is devaluing. The worker is not in the relationship from choice but is there because he/she is paid to be there; the relationship is circumscribed by this. But mental health workers do have an important role to play in sustaining other social relationships when these become strained by the difficulties associated with mental distress. Problems may arise from the behaviour of the individual, or they may result from negative assumptions and expectations, associated with mental illness, held by family and friends. Perhaps the success of a relationship between mental health worker and client might best be judged in terms of the extent to which it helps the client to maintain and regain other relationships of value.

Of great importance to people who face the challenge of recovery are relationships with others who have experienced similar difficulties. Others who have embarked on the journey of recovery are often more likely to inspire hope and offer pointers, role models and a vision of the future. It is vital that mental health professionals recognise

> *...the gift that people with disabilities can give each other...hope, strength and experience as lived through the recovery process...a person does not have to be 'fully recovered' to serve as a role model. Very often a person who is only a few 'steps' ahead of another person can be more effective than one whose achievements seem overly impressive and distanced.* (Deegan 1988)

Young & Ensing (1999), in their interviews and focus groups with people who had experienced serious mental health problems, remarked upon

> *...the tendency of people to speak primarily about their relationships with other people with psychiatric disabilities when discussing significant relationships in their lives. Although relationships with family members were mentioned by several participants, the majority reported that it was their relationships with other people with psychiatric disabilities that were the most meaningful and supportive.* (Young & Ensing 1999)

People may have contact with others in a similar situation directly, or via their writing (Deegan 1989, Spaniol & Koehler 1994, Reeves 1998, Kirkpatrick et al 2001): 'My suggestion is to get as many success stories from those who have schizophrenia to give a sense of hope to those just beginning their journey' (a participant cited in Kirkpatrick et al 2001). Others have found inspiration in accounts of people facing other challenges: 'I worked it out for myself by reading a lot about people in extreme situations, dying of cancer etc. and how they came through' (Pam, cited in *Roads to Recovery*, Mind 2001).

In mental health services there is a tendency to regard relationships as a 'one-way street'. Workers, friends and relatives give support and help, which the person with mental health problems receives. It is important to recognise that meaningful relationships are as much about giving as receiving. Always being on the receiving end of help is a dispiriting and devaluing experience. To reciprocate and to help others makes one feel valued and worthwhile.

Spirituality, Philosophy, Understanding

Typically, when we, as mental health workers, consider issues of understanding and acceptance we think in narrow terms about promoting 'insight' about 'illness'. What we often miss are the broader, philosophical, 'meaning of life'-type questions: 'Why me?' 'What is the point?' 'How can I understand what has happened to me?' Such questions are critical to understanding and accepting what has happened.

Deegan (1999) has emphasised that accepting 'illness', as such, is *not* part of the recovery process; however, coming to an understanding of what is happening that allows the person to take responsibility for themselves is key. Some people make sense of their experience in scientific terms, some see it in religious or spiritual terms, while others use social or psychological frameworks; there are many explanations of the 'meaning of life'. The critical issue is not whether such explanations are 'right' or 'wrong': believing in assorted neurotransmitters is not necessarily better than having faith in deities. Each person has to develop his/her own understanding, as it is rare for someone else's explanation to make sense to you without at least some modifications.

The critical question is whether an individual's understanding makes sense to him/her and at the same time allows the possibility of hope and growth. It is not possible to embark on a recovery journey if you believe that you are passively determined by someone or something else, whether this be inescapable fate, the unmodifiable action of genes, or all-knowing, all-powerful professional experts. Recovery involves active participation.

Taking Back Control

In recovery, self-determination is important: 'We are learning that those of us with psychiatric disabilities can become experts in our own self-care, can regain control over our lives, and can be responsible for our own journey of recovery.' (Deegan 1992).

The process of taking back control involves taking charge of your problems, i.e. learning what helps and what doesn't, learning how to live with the ups and downs, and learning how to protect yourself from things that make the problems worse. Mental health workers and others who have experienced similar problems can offer information about things that have helped and hindered others, but each person's situation is unique and each must find his/her own way of dealing with the problems encountered.

But taking control involves more than just dealing with problems. It means making decisions about your life and pursuing your interests. We may take advice from other people, but we must evaluate this advice ourselves rather than letting others make decisions for us. Enabling people to regain control does not, however, mean simply letting them get on with it; help and support are still important. Most of us rely heavily on the encouragement and assistance of others in order to be able to do the things we want to do.

Coping with Loss

Coping with the multiple losses that mental health problems can bring necessitates the processing of what has happened. Moving beyond hopelessness and despair necessarily involves a grieving process, but this does not follow some pre-determined sequence. Sometimes it is assumed that grieving and acceptance of loss must occur before a person can begin to move forward, but this is not necessarily the case.

Numerous accounts of recovery illustrate how the implications of mental health problems can initially be too much to grasp. Mental health professionals often see such denial as a problem, as an inherent part of the person's mental health difficulties that must be challenged before progress is possible. People who have been forced to rebuild their lives in the face of mental health problems often have a different perspective on this: they see denial as important in enabling them to keep going and retain hope in the face of catastrophic events.

> *I refused to believe I was crazy. I kept saying 'I have problems. I'm not crazy'. … It was denial internally that allowed me to go to school and do the things I needed to do to get a better life … (Donna, cited in Vincent 1999)*

> *They said to me there's no hope. And I said to myself 'No way' … It took years to accept it. What it would mean. And what it would have to do with my life … It took years. (Jennie, cited in Vincent 1999)*

Vincent (1999) explored the experience of people with mental health problems who had succeeded in obtaining good jobs. She concluded that denial can be important in enabling people to resist the stigma of a 'mental illness' label. It was only after people had started rebuilding their lives that they were able to move beyond denial to an acceptance of the need to address and manage their symptoms. Such a conclusion flies in the face of the accepted wisdom that people must gain 'insight' before they can move on. It suggests that, for many, the reverse is true: they can only begin to accept and face what has happened to them after they can see the possibility of rebuilding their lives. This makes sense. If all people know are the stereotypes, then acceptance of their mental health problems is terrifying:

> *All I knew were the stereotypes I had seen on television or in the movies. To me, mental illness meant Dr. Jekyll and Mr Hyde, psychopathic serial killers, loony bins, morons, schizos, fruitcakes, nuts, straight jackets and raving lunatics. They were all I knew about mental illness, and what terrified me was that professionals were saying I was one of them. (Deegan 1993)*

When someone has begun to see that their life can mean more than these stereotypes, then acceptance may be less difficult. However, such acceptance may still not be necessary. If people are able to rebuild their lives, does it really matter whether or not they believe they have mental health problems?

The Quest for Meaning and Value

Everyone needs a purpose in life, and striving to achieve meaning and value is central to the recovery process. 'I need to do something that makes me feel like I'm not just filling up space. I know for me I need to do something where I feel like I'm doing something important.' (cited in Young & Ensing 1999) What we do is central to the way in which we see ourselves and our relationships with others. In almost any social situation, one is first asked, 'What is your name?', followed by, 'What do you do?' Being valuable is important in counteracting despair. A sense of meaning and purpose fosters hope and the development of a positive sense of self. For many, satisfying work is central. However, meaning and purpose vary from person to person. Work is important, but it is not the only socially valued role. For some people other things are more valued: motherhood, politics, friendship, sports, environmental activism, church membership, drama, arts, voluntary work, education, and so on. However, most of these sources of value and purpose are a million miles away from the 'day-time activities' that are often recommended by mental health workers. The activities and roles from which most people with mental health problems derive meaning and purpose span the same range as for those who do not have such difficulties. How many non-disabled people find meaning and value in, for example, traditional 'occupational therapy' and the activities in 'day centres'?

That which is valuable and meaningful to an individual cannot be separated from that which is deemed meaningful and valuable in the communities and societies which they inhabit. Although there are many different ways in which people can contribute to the society in which they live, meaning and value are socially determined. If people with mental health problems are to be included in their communities they must have access to the valued opportunities within them.

RECOVERY: A CONTESTED CONSTRUCT

The concept of recovery has not been without its critics. Some commentators have misunderstood the term as something similar to 'cure' and have therefore argued that recovery is not possible for people whose problems are ongoing; they do not 'recover'. We believe that such arguments run counter to the user-defined model that we have developed here:

◆ Recovery is not an end-point but a continuing journey: people are not 'recovered', they are 'recovering'.

◆ Recovery is not the same as 'getting better': people are not recovering from illnesses, but recovering meaningful and valuable lives whether or not their problems can be eliminated.

Coleman (1999) has argued that professionals may view recovery as little more than maintaining a person in a stable condition. This is certainly not the model described here, which is about development rather than maintenance. However, it is important to remember that clinicians have been rather more pessimistic about people 'getting better' than the long-term outcome literature would indicate. In a review of seven long-term follow-up studies, Harding and Zahniser (1994) concluded that half to two-thirds of people significantly improved to the point at which they required no medications, were working, were integrated into the community, and were 'behaving in such a way as not to be able to detect ever having been hospitalised for any kind of psychiatric problem'.

Turner-Crowson and Wallcraft (2002) asked the question, 'Is there a danger that an over-emphasis on recovery could be an additional burden for people who do not feel they are in "recovery", whereas language such as surviving, coping, or developing strategies for living is more neutral and accepting?' However, they do go on to argue that, 'On the other hand, some find the concept of recovery inspiring and liberating, offering the prospect of going beyond simply "coping with distress"'.

We accept that the term 'recovery' may be open to misinterpretation, but the same may be true of any term. The recovery paradigm described here is founded in the accounts of those have themselves experienced serious mental health problems, and has already gained momentum within mental health policy and practice in the UK, North America, Australia and New Zealand. It has generally proved itself to be dymanic, inspiring and creative approach that can substitute hope for despair. It circumvents sterile arguments between competing intervention models (medication vs. therapy vs. employment vs. self-help vs. complementary therapy, etc.). All or none of these may contribute to the central, overarching, goal of growth and development. The highly individual nature of the recovery process means that different people will find different approaches helpful in the journey of rebuilding valued, meaningful and satisfying lives.

TOWARDS A MODEL FOR MENTAL HEALTH PRACTICE

If mental health workers are to inspire hope and promote recovery, then three interrelated components are central (see Fig. 4.1):

Developing hope-inspiring relationships

The presence of hope-inspiring relationships is an essential foundation for growth and development. It is not possible to regain the self-belief that is necessary for recovery in a relationship in which the 'patient' is dependent on the 'expert professional'. In developing a relationship that enables a person to move forward in life, the mental health worker's ability to inspire hope and self-confidence are of the essence. In building hope-inspiring relationships mental health workers must genuinely value and accept people for what they are; see and believe in their potential and abilities; listen to, accept and actively explore their experiences; tolerate uncertainty about the future; and help them to build on the problems and set-backs that will be part of their recovery processes. It involves a willingness to persevere and continue believing in someone even when everything seems to be going wrong, coupled with a genuine empathy and concern for their well-being, and a measure of humour – laughing with (not at or about) that person.

Facilitating personal adaptation: understanding, acceptance and taking back control

Helping someone to accommodate what has happened and move forward in life does not involve telling that person what to do. Instead, it is about inspiring the hope and confidence necessary to mobilise his/her internal resources, i.e. to use existing skills and develop any new ones necessary to pursue interests and ambitions. This involves enabling people to understand what has happened to them (in a way that both makes sense to them and allows them the possibility of growth), and helping them to develop ways of coping and taking control of their mental health problems and their lives.

Promoting inclusion: helping people to access the roles, relationships and activities that are important to them

Assisting people to maintain or rebuild satisfying lives involves facilitating engagement in roles, relationships and activities that are important to them. Such access is important in fostering and maintaining hope. It may involve helping people to access material resources (money, housing, decent clothing, possessions, etc.), assisting them to maintain existing roles and relationships and/or helping them to develop new ones, and facilitating engagement in valued activities. Maintaining and/or rebuilding roles, relationships and activities does not simply involve changing individuals so that they 'fit in', or helping them to develop the skills they may need. It also means ensuring that they have the necessary support, and helping them to negotiate any social and environmental changes that may be necessary in

order to facilitate access. Ideally, the mental health worker should try to promote the ordinary friendships, intimacies and social supports that can minimise the role that psychiatric services play in the person's life (Fig. 4.1)

It is these three dimensions of hope-inspiring competence that lie at the
heart of a model for mental health practice that can facilitate recovery.
However, these do not follow some set formula or sequence. It is not necessarily the case that mental health workers must first develop hope-inspiring
relationships and then move on in a stepwise fashion. For example, helping
people with practical things such as income/benefits, housing, and purpose-
ful activities can be important in the process of developing hope-inspiring

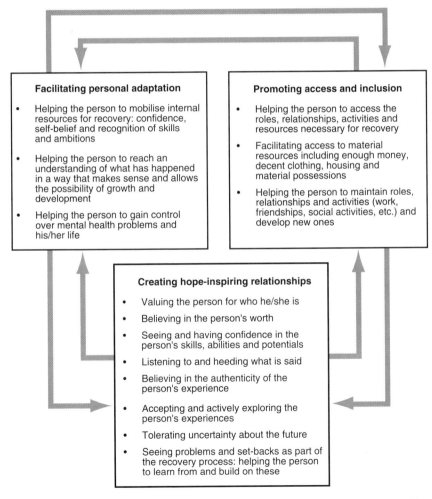

Figure 4.1. Social inclusion and recovery: components of a model for mental health
practice

relationships. Similarly, it may be that through beginning to do things that they value, an individual begins to develop confidence and gain control. A positive feedback loop can develop whereby increased confidence and control leads to greater success in developing meaningful roles and relationships, which in turn further increase confidence and hope.

Section 2

Facilitating recovery: promoting personal adaptation and adjustment

2

5

Barriers to relationship formation

INTRODUCTION

Responsibility for the development of effective, hope-inspiring relationships rests with the practitioner. Time and perseverance may be required. People with mental health problems have often had negative experiences of mental health services and the workers who inhabit them. Perhaps they have been detained in hospital against their will. Perhaps professionals have failed to listen to them, or have seemed unable to understand their situation and feelings. Even without such experiences, the prejudice associated with mental health problems may make many equivocal about using services.

Relationships of any kind are complex and fraught with potential problems. Because of the context in which they occur, relationships between mental health workers and clients are particularly susceptible to difficulties such as over-dependence and abuse of power. The aim must be to help people to overcome their difficulties and use their own resources in pursuit of their ambitions. Yet, in reality, practitioners too often tell people what they can and cannot (and should and should not) do, make decisions on their behalf, and pass judgement on their abilities and aspirations. There are many reasons for this. Barriers to the formation of constructive, hope-inspiring relationships arise from a number of sources: the circumstances in which the relationships are formed; the background, characteristics, beliefs and interests of those involved; the difficulties and disadvantages associated with mental health problems; and the attitudes of practitioners.

CONTEXT AND CIRCUMSTANCES: ISSUES OF POWER AND POWERLESSNESS

Relationships between mental health workers and those using services are, in many ways, different from those that occur outside the mental health arena. Unlike many relationships with professionals such as lawyers, mechanics, restaurateurs, physicians and surgeons, the relationship with a mental health professional involves people in discussion of their intimate feelings and personal areas of their lives and relationships: often things they have shared with almost no one else. But, unlike those relationships in which people usually share such intimate concerns – those with friends, partners, families – this exposure is a one-way process. One party talks of his/her thoughts and feelings, hopes and fears; the other does not. The relationship lacks the reciprocity of most intimate relationships because the role of 'helper' and 'helped' are clearly prescribed. The relationship may benefit both parties, but the way in which it benefits each one is quite different. The person is there because he/she, or someone, else considers that he/she has problems for which help is needed. The mental health worker is there because he/she is paid to provide such help. The 'helper' gains a salary for this help, together with those other benefits that employment can bring: job satisfaction, professional status, a sense of purpose, and personal achievement.

These power differentials may impede relationship formation. It is not uncommon for people with mental health problems to reject the approaches of mental health workers. It is often difficult to trust someone with your thoughts, feelings and experiences when they do not reciprocate: it can leave you feeling very vulnerable and exposed. It is difficult to believe that someone really cares about you when he/she is paid to be there. You also take the risk of being misunderstood – of your words being (mis)interpreted or analysed or judged. Mental health practitioners have traditionally spoken to 'their patients' in order to make a diagnosis, prescribe medication, assess changes in symptoms, and make decisions about their placement. It can be difficult to speak openly to someone who may translate your words and actions into diagnostic categories and treatment needs with which you may not agree.

Given the context of prejudice that prevails, a diagnosis of 'mental illness' offers an awful prospect. The mental health worker often embodies all that the client does not want to be, the help they do not want to need or believe that they require, and the services that they do not wish to use. The situation can be aggravated by compulsory hospitalisation and treatment. From the perspective of people so detained, the worker takes on the role of jailer, which makes a collaborative alliance difficult. The existence of compulsion affects power relationships between mental health workers and clients whether or not the service-user is compulsorily detained. This is particularly true in in-patient settings. As Campbell (1996a) explains:

> *That an individual can be compelled to receive psychiatric treatment affects each patient regardless of whether his [or her] stay is formal or informal. It is hardly possible to be unaware that you are being cared for within a legal framework which allows for treatment against your will.*

Because the possibility of compulsion exists, anyone using these services may feel wary of trusting mental health workers, being cautious about sharing their thoughts, feelings and experiences for fear that this may result in compulsory detention and treatment. In such a situation it is essential that mental health workers:

◆ recognise the privileged positions that they occupy
◆ acknowledge the power differentials that exist
◆ be aware of the difficulties that power differentials cause for those on the receiving end
◆ recognise that privilege does not render mental health workers 'superior'
◆ accept that, in a different place and time, workers could be on the receiving end themselves
◆ accord the person the dignity and respect that we would expect were the roles reversed.

DIFFERENCE AND DIVERSITY: BACKGROUND, CHARACTERISTICS, BELIEFS AND INTERESTS

Most people select, as confidantes, people who share their own values, beliefs and experiences (Fehr 1996). However, those using mental health services do not choose the workers whom they see. Because of this, mismatches between the characteristics, beliefs and interests of the practitioner and the client can impede the relationship between them. For example, the relationship possibilities between a young, white, graduate nurse and an older mother of three who emigrated to the UK from Jamaica are quite different from those existing between the same nurse and a young person who has just dropped out of university because of his mental health problems. Even where some choice of practitioner is possible, this choice is often very limited. Although efforts are being made to increase the diversity of mental health workers, it remains unlikely that the staff population will fully reflect the population using the services.

Mental health practitioners are all of working age and employed in jobs which afford them a certain status within society. Many have gained higher educational qualifications, have homes and families, and enjoy a range of leisure pursuits. Many people who experience mental health problems lack these advantages, and, in consequence, their lives and options are very different. Mental health practitioners often have all the ordinary things that those who use the mental health services have lost, or risk losing, as a consequence of their association with these services. Such differences mitigate against the formation of effective relationships. They influence the extent to which the practitioner can understand and empathise with the values, aspirations and problems of those with whom they are working. It is important that mental health workers recognise and address the differences that exist. They must acknowledge and explore how it feels to receive advice and help from someone who has opportunities that are not open to him/her.

It is also important that mental health workers are sensitive to issues of culture, ethnicity, class, sexuality and age. This must include an understanding and acknowledgement of the discrimination that people may have experienced within services and outside. Exploring the racism or homophobia/heterosexism that a person has experienced, and how that has affected his/her life is important in developing a relationship that will facilitate recovery.

However, as mental health workers we must also acknowledge what we do not know. Too often, in the face of something that we do not understand, we resort to inaccurate stereotypes: 'Work and education are more important to young men than to older women', 'Asians have supportive extended families', and so on. As everyone's experiences are different, we must explore each person's unique values and experience. But we can only know which areas to explore if we understand the things that may be important to people from different cultures and backgrounds.

For example, one young Caribbean woman with whom we worked was the only person from her family and social circle to have gone to university. She subsequently trained to be a social worker. While this may sound like an unqualified success story, it had resulted in numerous negative consequences in her life. Her friends and family did not really approve of her going to university. They believed that she saw herself as 'a cut above' them and was 'letting down' her community. She lost her boyfriend and many friends in the process, and relationships with her family became strained. When she became a social worker she was seen by some people as having become part of an oppressive 'establishment'. These difficulties were compounded when her mental health problems resulted in her losing her job and new-found friends. Her marriage broke down, she was evicted from her home, and her children were taken into care. She then felt utterly hopeless – that she belonged nowhere. She had lost both her former life and the new life that she had built for herself.

Awareness of cultural difference is equally important in relation to other facets of diversity. The experience of 'coming out' will undoubtedly have been a highly significant event for a lesbian or gay person and is likely to have had an impact, for both good and ill, on that person's life and relationships. Ignorance of the significance of the 'coming out' process not only mitigates against understanding, but can also have destructive consequences. For example, a person may not have 'come out' to his/her parents. If the mental health worker is unaware of this, he/she could cause problems by, for example, inadvertently 'outing' them to the parents against the client's wishes and thus jeopardizing family relationships.

Making use of the diversity that exists within a staff group can be helpful in informing the practitioner of issues that might be important. Staff members from different cultures and backgrounds can be important sources of information and expertise, but this resource can be utilised only if we are able to value the diversity that exists within the staff team and reduce the discrimination that exists within our services.

While increased diversity in the team may help improve understanding of different lifestyles, cultures and experiences, contradictory and competing values can impair relationships between mental health workers and with those who have mental health problems. For example, it would be difficult for a mental health worker with religious beliefs that declare homosexuality a sin to work with a gay colleague or to accept the aspirations of a gay client, helping him/her to access gay culture and supporting his/her homosexual relationships. It may be necessary for workers to suspend their own beliefs about what is right and wrong in order to help people rebuild their lives as they wish. There may also be times when mental health workers are unable to do this. Then they must be humble enough to question if they are really the best helpers for certain individuals. Sometimes another practitioner may be better equipped to work with a particular service-user.

DIFFERENCE AND DIVERSITY: MENTAL HEALTH PROBLEMS AND THEIR CONSEQUENCES

Although some efforts are being made to employ people with mental health problems (Sherman & Porter 1991, Perkins et al 2000, 2001a), it remains the case that most mental health workers have never themselves experienced life with mental health problems and the discrimination and disadvantage that accompany them. This is another difference that can form significant barriers in relationships.

Mental health problems may cause a person to behave in ways that seem incomprehensible to others, making them appear unreliable and unpredictable. Relationships can be jeopardised if, on some occasions, someone is pleasant and friendly, and on others, for no apparent reason, is abrupt or uncommunicative. There can be a real temptation to withdraw from that person completely. Most people with serious mental health problems have experienced situations in which their difficulties have led to the breakdown of friendships and relationships. Too often this means that the person must negotiate a frightening set of experiences alone, with no one there to understand and share their burden. The unrelenting negativity of someone who is depressed, the constant seeking of reassurance from someone who is anxious, and the jumbled thoughts and unshared perceptions of someone with a diagnosis of psychosis can all make relationships difficult. If someone believes things that no one else believes or is suspicious of those around them, then it is very difficult to form a relationship with him/her. But it is possible. The key to this possibility is understanding the person's own feelings and behaviour from within that individual's own frame of reference.

It is not simply cognitive and emotional problems that hinder relationship formation. The ways in which society responds to people who have these experiences are equally, if not more, important. The experience of discrimination which results in repeated rejection and exclusion can make a person understandably suspicious of forming new relationships. If everyone else has let them down, why should we, as mental health workers, be any different?

Adverse experiences of the mental health system can also impede relationship formation. It can be difficult to trust people who are part of a system within which the police have brought you to hospital as if you were a criminal, within which you have been restrained and forcibly medicated, and within which people have dismissed your views and wishes as merely symptoms of your madness. Mental health workers may have to do a great deal of bridge-building in order to demonstrate that they may be able to provide useful help and support to those who use such services. Such bridge building must start with understanding. If there are people within the staff who have themselves used mental health services, then these people can be a very valuable resource for assisting staff members who lack such experiences, though only if they are able to be open about these experiences. Prejudice and discrimination ensure that workers who have personal experience of mental health problems often keep very quiet about this (Anonymous 2001).

Given the discrimination that accompanies a diagnosis of mental illness, it is not surprising that people become angry, frustrated and aggressive. Aggression, and indeed violence, are a great impediment to relationships. If someone is aggressive towards us, our natural inclination is to avoid them, or fight back, or feel nervous or resentful of them. If aggression results from our attempts to be helpful then such feelings are likely to be even more acute. Aggression can make us feel inadequate. We are supposed to develop a trusting relationship with the person and help with his/her difficulties, but the rejection of help marks our failure to achieve this goal.

There is no easy way of dealing with such situations, and support from colleagues is likely to be essential, but we must use this support to try to understand why the client is behaving in that particular way. Admonishing the person for his/her 'inappropriate' or 'unacceptable' behaviour is likely to exacerbate the situation by demonstrating that we do not understand or empathise with his/her distress. The behaviour may be self-destructive or unacceptable, but it is understandable. We must demonstrate our understanding if we are to help people to find ways of living with what has happened to them.

ATTITUDES AND PRACTICES OF MENTAL HEALTH WORKERS

Reflection on our own practice, and the beliefs that underpin it, is as challenging as it is essential. It is very easy for all practitioners to harbour unhelpful attitudes and adopt practices that actively mitigate against the formation of relationships. We live in a world that devalues people who experience mental health problems. The fact that we work in mental health services does not make us immune to the attitudes that prevail in the communities in which we live. None of us can honestly say that we have always valued all those with whom we work. It is easy, from the best of motives, to behave in ways that are demeaning, but when we are really trying to do our best to help people it is easy to become defensive. This is problematic. As the *NHS Plan* (Department of Health 2000a) says 'The NHS needs to be seen to say sorry where things go wrong, rather than taking a defensive attitude, and to learn from complaints so the same problems do not recur.' If we are not able to be critical of ourselves then we cannot help those who may need our support. The error lies not in making mistakes, but in failing to learn from those mistakes.

Overzealousness and Blame

The primacy typically attached to cure means that mental health workers are often initially optimistic – perhaps over-optimistic – that people's problems can be eliminated. Such (over)–optimism is often shared by the client and by those close to the client; bewildered by what has happened, everyone hopes that everything will soon get 'back to normal'. However, when such expectations are not realised, it is easy for mental health workers to blame the client for 'failure' to improve, or to try to 'look after' him/her and take over his/her social roles.

These two responses constitute the 'high expressed emotion' which is a robust predictor of outcome (Vaughn & Leff 1976a,b, Bebbington & Kuipers 1994). Although such research was conducted in a family context it is important to note that the existence and consequences of high expressed emotion are not restricted to relatives. Both criticism and over-involvement are also found among staff who work with people who are experiencing mental health problems. Studies have found high levels of expressed emotion in around

40% of staff members working in both hospital and community settings (Kuipers & Moore 1995, Oliver & Kuipers 1996), and this forms barriers to the development of relationships that inspire hope and confidence.

It is not uncommon for mental health workers to become 'over-helpful', to make decisions for the person and to do things for him/her rather than supporting him/her to do things unassisted. This may result from simple lack of time on the part of the practitioners. It takes time to find out what a person wants, thinks and feels, how the client sees the problems, what he/she wants to achieve, and what help he/she wants. It can be so much quicker to make decisions for the person and do things for him/her. However, this has the consequence of diminishing the person's control and undermining his/her confidence and skills, thus impeding recovery.

'Over-helpfulness' may arise from the best of motives: from well-intentioned and successful endeavours to make sure that the client gets everything he/she needs. However, this may not facilitate recovery. If we have invested a great deal of time and energy in engaging that person, we may be reluctant to let go. We may come to believe that we are the only one who knows what that person needs and how to help him/her, and too often we also convince them that this is the case. Although it may be rewarding for us to see ourselves as someone's 'saviour' – the only one who is able to help that person – the dependence this attitude promotes is invariably destructive. The relationship is inevitably an unequal, abnormal and circumscribed one. It can never substitute for the range of reciprocal relationships that everyone needs. If the relationship between mental health workers and those whom they serve is to facilitate recovery then it must actively encourage the development of other roles and relationships rather than substitute for them. We can never do everything for someone, nor should we try.

The second feature of 'expressed emotion' – frustration, irritation and criticism – is equally evident among practitioners. Every mental health worker knows the feeling of pleasure when someone with whom we work does well. The person's success becomes an index of our own worth – a mark of our professional skill. This is not helpful. We may be able to act as a catalyst, but we cannot make a person recover, nor claim credit for that recovery. Recovery is something people do for themselves. There is a reverse side to this coin. Recovery is a 'rocky road' involving setbacks as well as progress. There will be times when people's problems get worse. If our sense of worth is dependent on continued improvement, then we all too easily become disappointed and angry when, despite our best efforts, the client does not make the progress we expected. We feel let down and may blame that person for 'lack of motivation', 'non- compliance', 'self-defeating behaviour', and 'failure to follow advice'. It is then tempting to withdraw – to try a little less hard. We must be able to see through our own frustration to that of the person we are trying to help if we are to be able to help them cope with the setbacks that are part of the recovery process. If we are to help people understand and accept such fluctuations of fortune, we must understand and accept them ourselves. Our task is to be there through the bad times as well as the good times, to 'stand by' people, and to believe in them when they have difficulty believing in themselves.

On the basis of the research into 'expressed emotion', Kuipers (2001) has outlined a number of things that help families to cope. These are probably equally important in enabling practitioners to cope.

◆ Finding something positive and likeable in the person
◆ understanding the difference between 'poor motivation' or 'laziness' and the difficulties that arise from the person's cognitive and emotional problems, thus reducing blame
◆ taking things gradually and building on small successes
◆ encouraging the person to develop and be as independent as possible
◆ maintaining a sense of perspective
◆ looking after ourselves.

Distancing

Regular contact with people who are extremely distressed and disabled by their mental health problems places great emotional demands on mental health workers. In a busy clinical situation it is often difficult to maintain an awareness of a person's feelings and needs and our own reactions to them. Distancing ourselves from the people with whom we work is one way in which we might try to protect ourselves. If someone behaves in ways that we consider unacceptable, or find disgusting, we may be tempted to emphasise the difference between us. It is very difficult to see them as 'like us', as a human being with adult sensitivities and feelings just like our own.

Such distancing is reflected in many of the practices in mental health facilities, especially in what might be termed the 'separates', i.e. separate staff crockery, cutlery, toilets and the like. Can there be anything more demeaning than being deemed unfit to use the same toilets as members of staff? The common justification for such practices reflects the 'them and us' barriers that prevail: 'they' do not have the same standards of hygiene as 'we' do. But can we really be fulfilling our duty of care if we expect people to use crockery, cutlery and toilets that are not sufficiently hygienic for us?

It can be embarrassing to take someone out when they smell unpleasant, or look strange, or talk loudly about inappropriate subjects. People stare. We feel demeaned by their assumption that maybe this is our brother, or our wife, or our father, or our friend. We may adopt various ways of distancing ourselves to make it clear that 'I am the professional, and they are the patient', that

'They're nothing to do with me, I'm just doing my job'. We might achieve this in a number of ways: by instructing them what to do and what not to do, in a loud voice; by leading them across the road by the hand; or by physically moving away from them or walking behind them.

Whether in public or in private, infantilisation (treating the person like a child) is one of the most common ways in which distance is achieved. When faced with someone who is unable to do the things that we expect of an adult, or unable to behave in the ways we expect of an adult, it is easy to fall into the trap of treating them as a child; a child cannot take full responsibility, may not be able to make decisions for themselves, must be protected, and must be taught the proper way in which to behave. Yet everyone knows how demeaning it is to be treated like a child. Far from inspiring confidence and hope, it saps self-confidence and self-respect. If a person is repeatedly treated like a child, is it any wonder when he/she ceases to take responsibility for what he/she does? Nor is it surprising if the person becomes angry with the worker (who may be many years their junior) who is infantilising him/her.

One of the major challenges facing any mental health practitioner is understanding why people behave in the ways that they do, and understanding that if they have lost all pride and hope, they may cease to look after themselves, bother what they do or look like, or care what others think. Distancing and infantilisation simply reinforce this hopelessness. If people are to develop self-respect and pride in themselves, then they need others (especially those mental health workers charged with helping them) to respect them. And there is always a great deal worthy of respect.

EXPERTISE AND GRATITUDE

Knowing things and having skills is good. There is nothing wrong with expertise *per se*, nor is there anything wrong with seeking confirmation of our expertise. It is the way in which this expertise is used, and the places in which we look to confirm it, that can be problematic.

Traditionally, it is assumed that mental health practitioners are the experts in mental health care. We use this expertise to tell people with mental health problems what to do to alleviate their difficulties. We expect the recipients of our assistance to respect our advice, to do what we tell them to do, and to be grateful for our help and assistance. Unfortunately, this approach is unlikely to facilitate recovery. As Barker (1992) cautions, 'We should not lose sight of the fact ... that the more useful we are, the more useless the person might become'. The world already tells people with mental health problems that they are useless. If practitioners in the services that are designed to help them confirm this by appearing to be the source of all knowledge, then they reinforce feelings of inadequacy and erode hope.

It is also the case that, if we, as practicioners, look to those whom we serve to confirm our expert status, we will tend to withdraw assistance from those who do not appreciate our advice. Many people who have mental health problems are 'sick and tired' of being told what to do, and may not want to take our advice. We are likely to feel affronted when they fail to take our pills, programmes and advice. Maybe we will decide that there is no point in them being here. We may as well discharge them because they are wasting scarce resources, better reserving our energy and efforts for those who appreciate what we have to offer.

Different people find different things problematic. Each person knows which of their cognitive and emotional problems is most troubling to him/her. If mental health workers cannot understand a person's difficulties from their own perspective then it is not possible for them to use their treatment and support skills to alleviate these problems. It is important that practitioners use their expertise to address those areas that are of most concern to the client, not simply those problems which the practitioners deem to be most important.

No support or treatment has the same effect on everyone who receives it. Research tells us about the average response of populations, in terms of both benefits and unwanted, unpleasant side-effects, but it does not tell us how an individual will respond. It is also the case that particular effects and side-effects may be valued differently by different people. For example, someone who finds his/her symptoms very distressing may be prepared to accept the sedating effects of a medication which reduces them. However, for someone whose symptoms are less intrusive, the same sedating effects might prevent that person from doing other things they want to do; the problems may outweigh the benefits. We can only know what is best for someone by asking him/her.

Even in ordinary, everyday situations when a person asks our advice ('Should I leave my boyfriend?', 'Should I telephone my mother?') we need to ask ourselves 'What are the consequences of giving this advice?' If we simply tell the person what we think they should do ('Yes, leave your boyfriend, he's no good for you.', 'No, don't call your mother, she only came to see you this morning.') then we may simply confirm for that person that he/she cannot make decisions for himself/herself and needs our expert guidance. There are other ways of responding, such as saying, 'I am not sure; what do you think?' and helping them think through the pros and cons of different courses of action. And there are also times when we must acknowledge that we don't know what's best. Sometimes we are reluctant to admit the limits of our expertise lest we lose our expert status. We might fall off our all-knowing pedestal, but this is no bad thing if it enables the client to believe that his/her own opinions are of value.

The challenge for mental health practitioners is to move away from a view of our 'professionalism' which dictates that we are the 'experts' and should tell people what to do, to one in which, as far as possible, we place our expertise at the disposal of those who need help. There will be limits, such as those imposed by mental health legislation, but there is also a great deal of latitude. There are always different ways of helping a person, i.e. many different drugs and therapies that could be used, and many different types of support that can be offered. We need to move to a position where we share our expertise with those whom we serve, and help them to decide what suits them best – even when this does not accord with our own judgements.

6

Creating hope-inspiring relationships

In most professional training, the ability to undertake therapeutic interventions – whether these be pharmacological, psychological or social – takes pride of place. However, such technical therapeutic competence can be effective only if we are also able to form supportive, hope-inspiring relationships with the people with whom we work. Such core relationship skills are equally important for practitioners who have professional mental health training and for those without such training.

In inspiring the hope that is essential for recovery, mental health workers face the twin challenges of appreciating the devastating impact of mental health problems on a person's life, and fostering a positive vision of future options. We must ourselves believe that everyone can grow within and beyond the limits of their problems if we are to foster this belief in others. Yet, if we focus only on future possibilities and fail to understand the often unpleasant reality of mental health problems, then we are likely to leave people feeling alienated and misunderstood. Encouraging exhortations such as, 'Don't dwell on that.' and 'It's all behind you now.' have a trite and somewhat hollow ring. On the other hand, dwelling on the difficulties that a person experiences at the expense of exploring the ways in which they can move forward also carries risks. The client is likely either to sink further into a spiral of despair, or to reject our negativity – and in so doing lose any support that we might be able to offer.

The traditional 'therapeutic triad' of empathy, non-judgemental warmth, and genuineness, described by Rogers (1957), has been elaborated and extended by a number of authors who have sought to define the skills and qualities necessary to develop effective therapeutic relationships (Perkins & Dilks 1992, Repper et al 1994, Perkins & Repper 1996, Coursey et al 2000). Service-users prioritise the values and attitudes of staff over skills (c.f. Repper 2000a). On the basis of questionnaires completed by over 500 people with mental health problems, Rogers & Pilgrim (1994) identified a number of qualities that were perceived as helpful. Most of these related to simple listening, and to the ordinary human qualities of empathy, tolerance, caring, and, most importantly, personal respect. Describing a nurse with whom a particular client had a positive relationship, one respondent said, 'She never talked down to me. She always treated me as an equal ...'.

Moving beyond focus groups and surveys of people's opinions, a number of authors have drawn on first-person accounts to define more specifically the attitudes and approaches necessary for the development of supportive, hope-inspiring relationships (Miller 1985, Woodside et al 1994, Russinova 1999, Kirkpatrick et al 2001). Valuing people, their hopes and dreams, understanding and accepting their version of events, believing in their skills, and helping them to pursue their own goals in life are all important. Also important in maintaining hope, however, is an appreciation of the nature of recovery – among both practitioners and those people making the journey.

VALUING PEOPLE AS HUMAN BEINGS

The ability to value the people as equals is central to effective relationship formation. If we are not able to see the people with whom we are working as our equals, and if we are not able to understand that, in different circumstances, they could be us or our nearest and dearest, then we cannot help them to develop and grow. It can be difficult to treat as equal someone who is behaving in unexpected, and perhaps unacceptable, ways – but it is vital. The ability to recognise the humanity of those with whom we work, value them and recognise the importance of their lives forms the essential bedrock upon which supportive, hope-inspiring relationships are based. An individual is much more likely to begin to value himself/herself if others value him/her. Deegan (1993) writes eloquently on this matter:

> There are people whose contribution we are able to see and value and there are those whose gifts we have failed to see and value... The real challenge in all this is to learn to value yourself. That can seem like such an impossible task because you get bombarded with messages and images that are so negative and degrading.

She goes on to reflect on what she would have liked to have said to herself as a 21-year-old who felt herself to be without worth and value.

> If I could reach back through the years I would hold you. I would say don't listen to the prognosis of doom ..... Don't give up ..... They may tell you that your goal is to become normal and to achieve valued roles. But a role is empty and valueless unless you fill it with your own meaning and

purpose .... You have the wondrously terrifying task of becoming who you are called to be .... Your life and dreams may have been shattered – but from such ruins you can build a new life full of value and purpose.

It is very easy for practitioners to endeavour to help people to grow and develop by emphasising what they *could become* without valuing who and what they *are now*. For everyone, future options are built upon accepting and valuing ourselves in the present. We need confidence now in order to build for a future, but in order to develop this confidence we need others to value us and to believe in us. Unless mental health workers can do this, hopes for the future cannot be inspired.

ACCEPTING AND UNDERSTANDING

Most people who have experienced mental health problems will too often have had their experiences dismissed by others, both within and outwith mental health services ('You only think that because you are ill, deluded...') When people relate strange and unusual experiences that others do not share, then it is easy to challenge them: to explain that they only think that because they are 'ill'. 'Delusion-busting' (Petch, personal communication, 2001) remains the norm in most mental health services: if someone says something that is manifestly 'untrue', then they should be encouraged to 'see the error of their ways'. Ironically, such an approach runs contrary to traditional psychiatric definitions of a delusion as a belief that is not susceptible to confirmation or disconfirmation by external events. If this were true, what would be the point of challenging delusions?

Recent cognitive models of thinking processes and perception argue that delusional beliefs are 'aspects of functioning not qualitatively different from normal processes but continuous with them' (Garety 1992). Moreover, as we have already described, the content of those beliefs defined as 'delusional' can often be significant. Even if it is assumed that 'delusional beliefs' have their origins in brain biochemistry, it is implausible that their content is also biochemically determined. It is not possible to believe that you are Jesus Christ in a society in which Christianity is unknown. The content of a person's beliefs is determined by their experiences and is thus critical in understanding the person. Willick (1992) writes of his son being 'plagued by the delusion that he has lost his heart' – a metaphorical interpretation of an emotional experience:

For many years before the onset of this delusion, Gary used other language to describe what he was experiencing. He said he couldn't get into anything, he couldn't get into his music, he was bad because he couldn't feel his previous affection for us .... So what Gary is saying is essentially correct – he has lost some of that capacity to feel strong emotions which all of us attribute, in our metaphoric way, to our heart, even though it is a function of our brain. We call it a delusion or false belief, although, in another sense, what he is saying is true – he has lost his heart. We accept it as a metaphor for his emotional experience; he experiences it in a concrete way with a literal meaning.

Most importantly, to deny another's reality prevents relationship formation. Any relationship, whether it be with partners, children, friends, or colleagues, relies on the ability of those involved to understand and share each other's world. Romme & Escher (1993) suggest that when faced with voice-hearers seeking help and support, we might ask ourselves to what extent the voices:

. . . indicate a sensitivity to other people's emotions or situations elsewhere (e.g. Gulf War)?
. . . relate to a stage of spiritual growth?
. . . reflect a destabilised identity resulting from either trauma or incomplete development?
. . . reflect recent or past traumas?
. . . reflect current emotional problems?
. . . reflect unfavourable current relationships or living circumstances?
. . . reflect interference with energies of a metaphysical nature?
. . . reflect illness, physical, physiological or psychological?

If practitioners see it as incumbent on themselves to 'correct' the 'misperceptions' of those defined as ill, then this simply serves to render people more isolated and alone. It is likely to increase despair ('No one will ever understand.') and thus actively impede relationship formation.

Not believing that I feel, see or hear the things that trouble me – that's what makes me really lonely. People say things like 'don't worry', 'it's in your imagination', 'of course no-one is talking inside your head and at your ears', 'it's just not happening'. Well all I can say to that is 'Yes, it is happening, more's the pity, and 'yes it is difficult' – but they don't understand. (woman with a diagnosis of schizophrenia cited in Perkins & Repper 1996)

In forming a relationship with someone who has ideas that seem strange and implausible to others – whether these are viewed as delusions or hallucinations, or construed as 'lack of insight' – it is important to start from the premise that everyone's construction of reality is different. It is impossible ever to say that we are 'right' and the other person is 'wrong'. Indeed there is no 'right' or 'wrong' just different ways of understanding what has happened that may be more or less useful, and more or less shared by others. As Romme & Escher (1993) conclude:

> *It is of little value to try to force a particular explanation upon someone; it should be recognised that other frames of reference may offer additional explanations, and in any case are likely to be sought out by the patient regardless of the therapist's personal insistence. Any frame of reference serves to order thought, and tends to encourage the desire to seek out a wider variety of explanations. Instead of sticking doggedly to some particular framework which may so far have been ineffective, it may be far more fruitful [for the therapist] to consider a number of other possible explanations.*

Perkins & Repper (1996) have argued that there are four important principles that apply to working with someone whose beliefs we do not share:

◆ Avoid trivialising or disregarding the individual. The beliefs that each person holds are real for him/her, whether or not they are shared by others. If someone denies or trivialises something that we hold dear, then it is difficult, if not impossible, to see that person as supportive and understanding.

◆ Take cultural factors into account. Not all belief systems can be subsumed under those of Western, industrial societies in which 'science' takes precedence over spirits, deities and supernatural powers. Even within one society, competing beliefs and values prevail: a 'wolf-whistle' may be seen as flattering by some readers and as unwanted sexual harassment by others.

◆ Explore the implications of the beliefs. A person's beliefs critically determine the way in which they feel and behave. It is a mistake to believe that because a belief is 'delusional' the person has no control over their behaviour. If, for example, I believe that you are trying to kill me, I have a range of options. I am not obliged to attack you; I could run away, lock myself up securely at home, give up, seek the protection of others, or report you to the police.

◆ Respond flexibly: there is considerable evidence that 'delusional' beliefs vary over time and according to the situation (Brett-Jones et al 1987), therefore the responses need to vary. When a person is questioning the veracity of his/her beliefs ('Is the food really poisoned?') then reassurance ('No it is not.') or contradictory evidence ('Well, everyone else is eating it, and it doesn't seem to be poisoning them.') may be effective. When the questioner is absolutely certain that the food is poisoned, such approaches are not likely to be effective.

Many people will have experienced their beliefs being repeatedly dismissed or invalidated by others, and may therefore have become reticent about sharing their feelings and experiences. The process of listening must be an active one; simply sitting there and making minimal responses – 'Yes.', 'Uh-uh.', 'How interesting.' – is unlikely to persuade that person that you are interested. If we are to understand their world, it is necessary to actively ask questions, explore what they are saying in their own terms and within their own framework. For example, if someone believes that they have committed a heinous crime, we might ask them what they have done, what happened, how they feel about it . . . .

BELIEVING IN THE PERSON'S ABILITIES AND POTENTIAL

The traditional focus of mental health services on deficits and dysfunctions means that it is very easy for both the client and those helping them to lose sight of that person's abilities and resources. If a mental health worker is unable to see the client's competencies and possibilities, then it is not possible for that practitioner to foster the hope that will enable the person to use these assets. If someone is to build a meaningful and valuable future, then his/her current skills must be the building blocks – the potential to be developed and exploited.

It can be hard to see beyond the multiplicity of difficulties that some people experience. Any assets may pale into insignificance in the face of what seem to be insurmountable problems. In such a situation it is very easy to fall into the trap of believing that nothing can be done until symptoms and problems have been alleviated. This is a mistake. First, the person's skills and abilities – including their tenacity and determination – are often critical in enabling them to overcome their symptoms and problems. Second, in order to engage with interventions and supports, people must believe that they have the resilience and resources necessary to build a better future. Third, there is never any guarantee that the various treatments and interventions available will significantly reduce someone's symptoms, so helping that person to do the things he/she can do in the presence of these symptoms may offer the only possibility of growth.

A very powerful example of the importance of focusing on strengths and interests rather than symptoms and treatments is provided by Mona Wasow's (2001) account of her son's progress:

> *In the old days, David's life consisted of sitting and staring into space, chain smoking, walking a lot, listening to his beloved folk music and coming home once a week for dinner. Today he still smokes and walks a lot, but he also works at a restaurant an hour a day, gets himself to a clubhouse for lunch everyday, and has learned to ride the buses so that he can get to his music and pottery lessons every week . . . . I do not believe these changes came about because of the possible tendency for schizophrenia to improve over the years. Nor do I believe that the newer medications played a role, since he had been taking them for many*

years before these positive changes occurred. David's changes came about rather quickly when professionals and family members began to focus on his considerable strengths instead of his illness . . . . In the old days the emphasis on his treatment, aside from medication was put on helping with his abysmal 'daily living skills' – helping him learn to ride the buses, to take a shower, to make eye contact and so on. But where should he go on the bus? For whom should he have a shower? With whom should he make eye contact? . . . This approach got nowhere. A few years ago . . . the psychiatrist said 'I don't want to hear all that again. That's his illness, and we have not been able to change that for years. Tell me about his strengths; we would do better to work on those.'

If a person simply waits until symptoms have subsided to a point at which he/she can start to use his/her abilities, then there could be a very long wait. Everyone knows how difficult it is to do something one has not done for some time; the longer leave it, the harder it gets. This is particularly so for social activities: if contact is not maintained it can be extremely difficult to pick it up again. Too often, social networks are eroded as contact with mental health services continues (Holmes-Eber & Riger 1990). This means that helping someone to resume activities as soon as possible, and to maintain social contacts, is essential.

Mental health practitioners have most difficulties identifying the assets of those with whom they find it most difficult to work. 'Difficult patients' are often people who are characterised as 'manipulative' and 'attention-seeking' or having 'personality disorder' rather than 'mental health' problems (Breeze & Repper 1999). In such situations it may be important to look at the not inconsiderable skills that those clients employ in their 'manipulative' or 'attention-seeking' behaviour. For example, one woman with whom we worked was described as continually interfering with what others were doing, and pestering the staff. These 'skills' were eventually exploited by giving her responsibility for a number of aspects of running the unit, such as keeping the notice-boards up to date, filing information, and taking minutes at meetings – positive and constructive ways in which she could 'interfere', and gain attention.

Identifying abilities is important in inspiring hope, but hope relates to the expectation that something meaningful to the individual can be achieved. The person's priorities and interests are therefore key.

ATTENDING TO PEOPLE'S PRIORITIES AND INTERESTS

Within mental health services, tension often exists between the priorities of mental health workers and those who use the services. The things which staff members deem to be appropriate and those which the person wants to achieve can be very different. From the best of motives, mental health workers identify things that they think would be 'good for' people, e.g. particular forms of therapy, activity or skills development (Shepherd et al 1995). If a person fails to adhere to these prescriptions, whether they be pharmacological, psychological, occupational or social, he/she is too often deemed to 'lack motivation' or to be 'non-compliant' (Chamberlin 1988).

If mental health workers are to foster supportive, hope-inspiring relationships, then people must see these as being able to help them with things that they want to achieve. If people can see nothing in it for them, then 'engagement' becomes less a collaborative alliance and more an interchange between warring troops engaged in a battle for supremacy (Campbell 2000). There are clearly circumstances in which a practitioner cannot accede to all of the person's requests, e.g. enabling him/her to obtain 'street drugs' or to leave hospital if that person is compulsorily detained. However, there are many other occasions when the limiting factor is no more than the mental health worker's belief that he/she 'knows best'.

An effective relationship involves mutual respect. This means that practitioners must be willing to accede to the wishes and priorities of those people with whom they work, even when these do not accord with what the mental health workers think is best. A person may prefer one type of drug, therapy, or support; if the mental health worker insists that he/she accepts another option, there is a risk that the person will reject any help at all. Acceding to someone's wishes, or negotiating a mutually acceptable compromise, is likely to foster a collaborative working relationship in which that person feels heard and valued; this therefore increases the likelihood of the individual accepting help.

Similarly, mental health workers may feel that some of the person's aspirations and ambitions are ill-founded. Perhaps we think that a person is not yet ready to get a job, or to embark on a university course, or that it is inadvisable for them to go out 'clubbing' with friends. In such a situation, it is tempting to try to persuade the person of the error of his/her aspirations, and to list the problems that may ensue if he/she embarks upon them. But to do so risks reducing that person's confidence and diminishing their enthusiasm and hope. Alternatively, the person may reject the practitioner's advice and help altogether, and carry on regardless – but with a greater chance of experiencing precisely those problems that the practitioner warned of, because of the absence of support.

Rather than advising against a particular course of action, the mental health worker could engage with the person's interests, help them to evaluate the possible benefits and costs, and work with him/her on ways of maximising the chances of success. For example, in relation to employment, even if we do not think that the person is ready to get a job, it is still possible to help him/her to look at what is available, fill in application forms, prepare for interviews and to support that person's efforts to keep the job if he/she is successful. With such support it is possible that the practitioner will be proved wrong: this is precisely the sort of help which research demonstrates can maximise people's chances of success (Bond et al 1997, 2001). If the person is not successful, then, by providing help, the mental health worker remains engaged with him/her, and is therefore able to help them to learn from the experience and explore different ways of achieving the goal.

It may also tempting for practitioners automatically to deny a person's request for help with something that he/she appears to be able to do unaided. It is generally argued that to provide help in such circumstances would be to de-skill that person and render them dependent. Yet there may be other, equally important, considerations. Asking for help is often a very difficult thing to do. To reject a request for help may be seen as a further rejection that demonstrates the practitioner's lack of understanding ('You're no help, you never do anything useful.'). To accede to people's wishes may be important in relationship-building, helping them to believe that there may be something in the relationship for them, and to feel heard and heeded, i.e. a partner in the relationship rather than the one who is always told what is best.

It may also be the case that the person is right, and the practitioner wrong, about the level of support needed. The possibility of relieving a person of some responsibilities in order to enable that individual to do other things that he/she values should not be overlooked. For example, a person may be able to travel to college or engage in a class, but may find doing the two things at once more than he/she can manage. In such a situation, it may be sensible for the mental health worker to relieve the person of responsibility for getting to the college, by arranging for an alternative form of transport so that he/she can do the course desired. It could be argued that the person should learn to travel on the bus before thinking about taking a course. However, there are problems with this. Travelling on a bus is not valuable to a person in and of itself, but is a means to an end. It is likely that the course is what that person values, and that success in this will be what gives him/her the greatest a sense of achievement (not to mention social contacts and valuable skills/qualifications). But, if we insist that the person learns to get there independently first, there is a risk that the he/she will give up on both: neither become confident in using the bus, nor undertake the college course, thus further eroding his/her hope and self-belief.

ACCEPTING FAILURES AND SETBACKS AS PART OF THE RECOVERY PROCESS

It is relatively easy to remain hopeful when everything is going well. The bigger challenge is to maintain a positive vision of the future when setbacks and disappointments occur. Fluctuating difficulties are unfortunately characteristic of many people with mental health problems. If each downturn is not to be a cause of despair, it must be anticipated and accommodated as part of the recovery process. It may not be possible to prevent relapse completely, but it is usually possible to identify early warning signs and minimise the disruptive consequences for the person's life. If people are able to identify when things are not going well, then there are a number of options. Perhaps they can cut down on activities and responsibilities, reducing the stresses in their lives. Perhaps some extra support may be enough to help them carry on. If this is ineffective, then taking time off sick is generally less disruptive than failing to do what is expected or behaving in ways that may be seen as inappropriate and disruptive. When things are getting better, extra help may be needed for them to get back into the swing of things. It may be helpful to ease back gently, with reduced duties, hours and responsibilities. The important thing is to make plans in advance for the ups and downs that will inevitably occur.

Even without the added complication of mental health difficulties, there are few people whose lives are always smooth. Difficulties and disappointments are facts of life; they sap self-confidence but may more readily lead to hopelessness and despair if a person has mental health problems. First, ordinary everyday difficulties can trigger an increase in symptoms. Second, ordinary stresses and strains exacerbate the lowered self-confidence that so often accompanies mental health problems. Third, it is tempting for people, and those around them, to mistakenly pathologise ordinary reactions to life events, attributing perfectly rational emotions (e.g. sadness about a friend's illness, or anxiety about a child's problems at school) to their mental health problems, perhaps concluding that they are unable to meet the demands of the situation. Finally, people who have experienced mental health difficulties may be relatively socially isolated and lack the ordinary supports upon which most of us rely so heavily when we experience difficulties.

Whether as a consequence of fluctuating mental state and its social and psychological sequelae or of the vicissitudes of everyday life, the fact that recovery does not proceed in an ascending linear fashion is one which both the person and those around him/her must accommodate. However, equally challenging is the fact that no one can know where the recovery road will lead.

ACCEPTING THAT THE FUTURE IS UNCERTAIN

Questions like 'Will I ever get better?', 'Will I ever be able to get a job, find a place of my own?', and 'If I have children, will they have mental health problems?' have been asked by the vast majority of people who have experienced mental health difficulties. People want to know what the future holds for them, and the answer is that practitioners do not know. The future is uncertain.

Many people with mental health problems think professionals have all the answers – and professionals often feel obliged to provide them. But when a person asks questions such as these it is easy to fall into one of two extremes. On the one hand, practitioners may try to be encouraging by saying things like, 'I'm sure you'll get better, get a flat, a job'. Such an approach is unlikely to be reassuring for people whose problems have continued for a number of years, during which time they have seen little progress towards the things they wish to achieve. On the other hand, in an attempt to help someone accept the 'reality of the situation', practitioners may look to population outcome data and provide answers in terms of the statistical (un)likelihood of that person ever being free of problems and achieving the things he/she wants to do. A strategy like this is likely to promote hopelessness.

Although population statistics may indicate the probability of a person, for example, getting a job, they do not tell us what the future holds for a particular individual. Opportunity and resources – both material and social – are important, but success is also dependent on the extent to which individuals believe in their abilities and on their determination to succeed. There is evidence from the employment field that personal and psychiatric variables are relatively unimportant in determining whether people will be successful in getting jobs (Secker et al 2001). The more important determinants are the type of support available, the extent to which a person wants to get a job, and that person's confidence in his/her own ability to work. People are more likely to be successful if they access jobs they really do want to do, or move into accommodation of their own choice, rather than those which professionals think are suitable for them (Chamberlin 1988).

Self-confidence and determination are strongly influenced by a person's belief in the possibility. This does not necessarily have to be founded on 'concrete, real-world evidence' but depends instead on 'a sense of the possible': a *belief* in personal competence, ability to cope, meaning and purpose, and well-being (Miller 1992). This 'sense of the possible' does not occur in isolation, but requires that others share in the belief. Instead of simply quoting gloomy statistics, mental health workers can honestly say that although it may be more difficult for someone with these problems to, for example, get a job, many people have succeeded in doing so. They can then go on to talk about the things that tend to make success more likely, and explore ways of circumventing potential barriers.

This positive and constructive accommodation of uncertainty is equally important in relation to the course of a person's problems, and it is important that the linkage between the presence of symptoms and the likelihood of achieving personally meaningful goals is not overstated. There is a multitude of examples of people being able live independently, work, raise children, and form relationships in the presence of a range of quite severe cognitive and emotional problems. The important issue is not usually the presence or absence of such 'symptoms' but the way in which the person accommodates and manages them. Many people find others' accounts of ways of coping (see, for example, Leete 1989) both helpful and hope-inspiring (Kirkpatrick et al. 2001).

In developing supportive, hope-inspiring relationships, practitioners must strike a delicate balance between optimism and realism. They must help people to overcome the doubts they may have in their abilities, while at the same time providing assistance in accommodating their problems. This balance is illustrated in the experience of one of the authors (R.P.) of this book.

I had been off work with mental health difficulties for several months and had lost confidence in my ability to return. I doubted whether I would be able to do my job. My psychiatrist was understanding and sympathetic. She said that I should not go back to work until I felt ready – really able to cope. I clearly did not feel confident about my ability to manage and this was confirmed by my psychiatrist saying that I should not go back to work until I did feel confident – therefore I concluded that I was not fit to work. And, as the weeks ticked by my confidence progressively decreased. Fortunately, one of my friends had a greater belief in me than I had in myself. Seeing what was happening she came to see me and was quite directive and apparently 'unsympathetic'. Or perhaps it would be more accurate to say that her sympathy and understanding took a different – and more constructive – form than that of my psychiatrist. She told me that the longer I stayed off work, the more difficult it would be to return. She effectively made me set a date for going back – but also recognised the very real difficulties I would have: she helped me to plan how I would prepare to go back to work – from negotiating with the occupational health physicians, to getting some work sent home so I could catch up with what I had missed, and meeting colleagues – and then gave me a lift in on my first couple of days back. Without such active confidence and encouragement I may never have returned to my job and my life today, more than a decade later, would be very different.

Balancing optimism and realism in this way involves taking risks. Given the focus on homicide and suicide of the last decade, professionals have understandably become more risk averse. This reluctance to take risks often goes well beyond issues of physical safety to encompass an avoidance of the risk of failure. The logic runs that people with mental health problems have often experienced many failures, which have eroded their self-esteem. Further failures must therefore be avoided as these would further diminish their confidence. But, in order to achieve anything a person must take risks;

the only way of avoiding failure is never to do anything. No mental health workers would be in their positions had they not taken risks: the risk of not passing exams, of not getting jobs when they applied for them, of not being able to do the jobs once they had got them, not to mention the myriad risks involved in all their relationships and commitments outside work. A focus on avoiding the risk of failure means never having the possibility of those successes which reinforce and promote confidence and hope.

Clearly, it is important that people understand the risks that they are taking, but, the bottom line is that *they* must decide whether a risk is worth taking or not. It may also be sensible to think about 'Plan B' – what you will do if you are not successful. However, confidence and preparedness to take risks interact. A person whose confidence is at a low ebb is less likely to take risks because he/she is pessimistic about the likelihood of success. It is always easier to take risks from a secure base, in the knowledge that someone will be there for you if things do not work out. The presence of someone in your life who believes in you and supports you in trying to do what you want to do – but who you know will be there, still believing in you, if you are not successful – can inspire the confidence needed to risk the possibility of success. A mental health worker can both support such relationships that already exist in a person's life, or provide a supportive, hope-inspiring relationship when this is lacking.

FINDING WAYS OF SUSTAINING OUR OWN HOPE AND GUARDING AGAINST DESPAIR

Hopelessness breeds hopelessness. If practitioners cannot see a positive future for those people with whom we work, then it is very easy for us to become 'burned out', hopeless and unable to see the point in what we are doing. This is particularly likely when we have too much to do and lack the time or resources to help people in the ways we know we could. It is all too frequent for our efforts not to be recognised by the organisation for which we work, or by the society in which we live.

In order to guard against our own despair, it is important that we organise support for ourselves. We cannot look to service-users to support us – we have to look elsewhere. Most of us gain a great deal of informal support from our colleagues, but we also need the more protected setting of supervision in which to review what we are doing, examine our feelings and reactions, explore the expectations we have of ourselves, and identify what we do well and what we need to work on. Effective supervision is essential for every mental health worker. It serves to sustain our interest and enthusiasm and develop our skills. It also enables us to address those broader questions about what we are doing and why we are doing it.

It is not only people with mental health problems whose hopefulness depends on a sense of meaning and purpose. Our own hope and commitment as mental health workers requires that we, too, have a clear understanding of the meaning and purpose of our efforts. In this context, the models that guide our work are particularly important.

Within traditional cure-based approaches we judge our skills and worth on the basis of the extent to which we are able to reduce people's problems. If, despite our best efforts, we are unable to get rid of a person's symptoms, a cure-based perspective is of little help in telling us what else we might usefully do. It is therefore all too easy for us to feel hopeless and give up, and if we give up hope, then we can only engender hopelessness in those whom we are trying to help.

A similar problem exists with the various skills-based approaches that have been developed (see Anthony, 1977 1979). These start not by thinking about symptoms and cures, but by focusing on skills and skills deficits and the ways in which people can be assisted to develop the competencies they need. Like cure-based approaches, the focus of skills models is on changing people so that they can fit into the world. Within this framework, we judge our abilities on the basis of whether we can help people to acquire the skills they need in order to fit in and live independently. If they need ongoing support and help – we again see ourselves as failures.

While symptom reduction and skills development have their place in a recovery framework, they do not constitute its guiding principles. Recovery is about rebuilding a meaningful and satisfying life, whether or not there are ongoing or recurring symptoms and problems, and whether or not the skills necessary to do everything independently have been acquired. Recovery is not about independence, it is about interdependence – about ensuring that people have access to the supportive relationships they need. Within such a framework, access and inclusion become more important than symptoms and skills. There are a wide variety of ways in which we can help people to develop the confidence and hope necessary to begin to explore their options, and there are numerous ways in which we can support these explorations. These involve not only, or even mainly, changing the individual to 'fit into' to an 'able-minded' world. Rather, they involve changing the prejudices and assumptions of that world, changing its capacity to accommodate people who experience mental health difficulties, and changing the support available to enable people to meet expectations and fulfil their ambitions.

A recovery perspective opens up a whole range of opportunities and possibilities for both the practitioners and those people who are experiencing mental health problems. If we are to take advantage of these opportunities, we must move beyond the boundaries of mental health services and accept the need to grow and develop ourselves.

ACCEPTING THAT WE MUST LEARN AND BENEFIT FROM EXPERIENCE

At the heart of our ability to establish supportive, hope-inspiring relationships is our continuing ability to learn from those whom we have the privilege of helping. Nowhere is this more essential than when we are having difficulties, as when our relationships with service-users break down or fail to get going in the first place. When this occurs it is important that we:

◆ recognise when there are problems in the relationship
◆ examine and reflect on our own feelings and expectations of both ourselves and of the person with whom we are working
◆ try to understand what the situation looks like, not from where we stand, but from the standpoint of that person
◆ examine our own behaviour and ask questions such as, 'How might what we said and did look to the person on the receiving end?', 'Why did we behave in the way we did?', and 'Were there other things that we could have done?'

For example, when someone refuses to see us, is hostile towards us, we must ask questions about what is generating this hostility and how we might be contributing to it; we must try to understand the person's antipathy towards us. Perhaps they resent us having a job, a home, status, all of which they so badly want. Perhaps we have failed to acknowledge, and be honest about, our privileged position. Perhaps they simply resent yet another person telling them what to do. Perhaps we have failed to recognise their abilities and have ridden roughshod over their wishes and ambitions. Perhaps they are suspicious that we, like so many other people in their lives, will let them down, infantilise them, and fail to understand their lives and experiences. Perhaps anger and hostility are the only ways in which they can share what has happened to them. The possibilities are manifold.

Having explored why the person may have responded to us in a particular way, it is then incumbent on us to explore different ways of behaving. Perhaps we should apologise for upsetting them, and ask what it is that has offended them. Perhaps we should ask them what they would find most useful. Perhaps we need simply to witness their anger and despair, and understand the bitterness they feel about what has happened to them.

We, as professionals, can learn more from the people with whom we work than we ever can from training and courses. But we can only learn if we 'swallow' our professional pride and hear what it is like to be on the receiving end of our ministrations. The process of such learning can itself contribute to the formation of supportive, hope-inspiring relationships because it requires us to respect the experience and opinions of the people with whom we are working. Flexibility, openness, and a willingness to be corrected by experience are essential if mental health workers are to facilitate recovery.

7

Facilitating personal adaptation: understanding and acceptance

INTRODUCTION

Building on the foundation of supportive, hope-inspiring relationships, the challenge of recovery may involve a number of components. Wing & Morris (1981) have argued that the extent to which someone with mental health problems is disabled is a function of three factors:

◆ The cognitive and emotional difficulties which lead to the diagnosis of mental health problems

◆ The social disadvantages that the person faces. These include pre-existing disadvantages (arising from things such as racism, poverty, poor housing, poor education, and disrupted family relationships) and also those that are a consequence of the prejudice and exclusion that accompany mental health problems. Such social disadvantages continue even if symptoms disappear: a history of mental health difficulties can be as disabling as their continued presence.

◆ The way in which the person understands and accommodates what has happened to them. The ways in which they cope with, or respond to, the cognitive/emotional difficulties and social disadvantages that they face.

If, as Wing & Morris (1981) suggest, disability is a consequence of clinical, social and personal or psychological factors, then the ways in which recovery might be facilitated can be understood on each of these dimensions:

◆ Clinical Recovery relates to the cognitive and emotional problems that a person experiences. Coleman (1999) has described 'clinical recovery' as the reduction or eradication of symptoms by treatment. Clinical recovery might also include the various ways in which people develop in order to accommodate and take control of their cognitive and emotional problems, and the ways in which they minimise the disruptive impact of these difficulties. These facets of recovery will be addressed in Chapter 8.

◆ Social recovery relates to the reduction of the social disadvantages that people face, and to the extent to which they are able to circumvent such barriers in order to access the roles, relationships and activities that they value. These facets of recovery will be addressed in Chapters 10 and 11.

◆ Psychological adjustment refers to the way in which people understand and accommodate the problems and disadvantages they face, described by Davidson & Strauss (1992) as the 'dawning of an awareness of a sense of self beyond one's illness'. Spaniol & Koehler (1994) have described how:

> *'Mental illness, and the negative personal and societal attitudes surrounding mental illness, often leave [the person] disconnected from themselves, from others, from their environment, and from meaning and purpose in life.'*

It is towards rediscovering a sense of self and facilitating personal adaptation and adjustment that this chapter is directed.

WAYS OF ACCOMMODATING A DIAGNOSIS OF MENTAL HEALTH PROBLEMS

Many people have described the ways in which they have sought to accommodate the experience of mental health problems and its consequences. These accounts show us that there is no single, optimal way in which this might be achieved: different approaches make sense to different people.

In Chapter 2, we described the ways in which popular portrayals of mental health problems offer an unenviable set of options. People are portrayed either as vulnerable, incompetent and unable to look after themselves, or as unpredictable and dangerous, or both. Either way, it is typically assumed that an ordinary life – a home, a job, a partner, children, a social life – is not a realistic possibility for someone with mental health difficulties.

Wing & Morris (1981) and Shepherd (1984) have described two common 'adverse personal reactions' to the experience of mental health problems that might loosely be described as 'denial of difficulties' and 'giving up'. Although these responses have been described as 'adverse', they may represent rational and adaptive ways of carrying on in the face of seemingly insurmountable problems. As we have seen, given the prevailing images of madness, it is hardly surprising that some people cope with the experience by denying that they have any problems at all ('I'm not like them', 'I'm not mad', 'There's nothing wrong with me.') and reject the services that have so defined them. In 'denial', people protect themselves from the prejudice and discrimination associated with using mental health services. They free themselves from clinicians' pessimistic prognostications that sap hope and self-confidence. But in rejecting assistance from mental health services, they may fail to obtain the help and support they may need to do the things they want to do. Their cognitive and emotional problems may also lead them to behave in ways that are considered 'inappropriate'. This may lead to their being excluded anyway, perhaps being labelled 'bad' instead of 'mad'. If their behaviour is deemed unduly disruptive or dangerous, then attempts to avoid contact with services may be thwarted by compulsory detention and treatment, with all the degradation and increased discrimination that this entails.

At the other end of the spectrum, it is equally easy for a person to give up completely ('I'm useless', 'Everything is hopeless', 'Nothing I can do will make any difference', 'What is the point?'): '. . . "giving up" apathy, and indifference become a way of surviving and protecting the last vestiges of a wounded self.' (Deegan 1990). On the positive side, 'giving up' protects people from the enormous challenges and from the high risk of failure inherent in the unequal odds they face. They also avoid undue stress that may make their problems worse. On the other hand, as they do less and less, their confidence and self-belief are further eroded to the point at which even the smallest everyday tasks become major challenges. By 'giving up' people are unable to make the most of their abilities or avail themselves of opportunities to move forward. It is important to emphasise that these responses are not an intrinsic part of a person's mental health problems. They are ordinary, understandable ways in which people cope with a range of devastating life events.

Hatfield & Lefley (1993) describe a number of other ways in which people faced with the challenge of living with serious mental health problems have accommodated their experiences. One man argued that to have a mental illness is unfair, but then life is unfair – in different ways to different people. He accepted his problems, but rejected bravado as a way of coping with the pain and humiliation, seeing this as a denial of 'the almost heroic reality, that the strength to endure and overcome had to arise as a strategic reaction to an unchosen, unforseen misfortune.' (Weiner 1987). Another argued that 'life puts various limitations on all people, but freedom to choose always exists within these limitations' (cited in Hatfield & Lefley 1993). Perhaps more fatalistically, Pilvin (1982) concluded that the experience of mental health problems 'made me understand that there are no guarantees, that the outcome of my plans may be beyond my control.'

Many authors talk about the importance of acceptance as the basis for recovery: the value of accommodating what has happened in order to move on. The rekindling of hope is a key component of this: people can only accept their situation if they believe they will be able to cope with that situation, and can embark on the journey of recovery only if they have the hope that it might lead somewhere (Deegan 1996). Hope takes different forms for different people. Some people find that hope lies in the belief that a cure will be discovered. The continued search for a cure has been a motivating force in the lives of many people. As well as the various physical and pharmacological remedies of traditional medicine, people with both physical difficulties (see, for example, Picardie 1998) and cognitive/emotional problems (see, for example, Faulkner & Layzell 2000) have explored the range of 'complementary' and 'alternative' remedies that are available. While the search for the resolution of difficulties may provide a purpose and meaning in life, it can mean that people's impairments, or rather the quest to eliminate them, take over their lives completely, replacing all other goals and ambitions.

Others have sought a broader sense of meaning and purpose that goes beyond their problems. For some people, this involves minimising the significance of their impairments – relegating them to a small and insignificant corner in an attempt to 'be positive and try to get on with life' (Anonymous 2001). Hope for this person, as for many others, is firmly rooted in pursuing a range of work, social and personal goals in which mental health problems play no part. The person quoted, who had a diagnosis of schizophrenia, chose to remain anonymous rather than being identified as someone with schizophrenia. There are numerous accounts of people making this decision not to 'come out' about their mental health problems (Dunn 1999) and there are many reasons for choosing not to do so.

Clearly, prejudice and discrimination may be a major motivation for not telling others about your mental health problems. If you say that you have such difficulties, many employers will not hire you, many colleges and training courses will not accept you, and other people may avoid you or treat you differently. One woman told us how she had got talking to a man in a pub and had eventually 'let slip' that she had been in a psychiatric hospital 'soon after that he said he was going to the loo . . . and never came back again.' Avoiding discrimination and rejection are undoubtedly a very powerful reason for keeping mental health problems hidden, and this can be an effective strategy to enable one to do the things one wants to do.

It is obviously easier for people to keep quiet about their mental health problems if they can hide them. While this is possible for some, it is less easy for those whose behaviour may sometimes be influenced by their difficulties. Even if this is the case, it is still possible for people to minimise the importance or significance of their difficulties. There are many with visible mobility/sensory impairments who have adopted this approach: although President Roosevelt could not stand or walk unaided, he never talked about, or dwelt upon, these difficulties. People with mental health problems who cope by minimising their difficulties tend to reject the pity that having such problems often attracts; they see it as an insult to their strength and competence. They also tend to reject a more radical 'user'/'survivor' role, seeing this a distraction from the other more important roles that give their lives meaning and purpose (e.g. as a worker, politician, father, tennis player, etc.).

However, there are an increasing number of people with mobility/sensory and/or mental health problems who actively and positively embrace these features, seeing them as central and important parts of their identity alongside their other identities. People who adopt this type of approach take a pride in a user/survivor or disabled-person identity and celebrate the contribution that they can make because of, not in spite of, their experiences. Such a perspective can be seen in many parts of the Disability Movement and, within the mental health arena, in organisations such as Survivors Speak Out and Survivors' Poetry, which developed in the 1980s, and in the Mad Pride movement that emerged in the latter part of the 1990s (Curtis et al 2000). People like Peter Campbell (1996a,b) in the UK and Judi Chamberlin (1977) in the USA, to name but two of many, have had important political roles as activists in the world of mental health. As part of wider movements, such individuals have made an important contribution to an understanding of the situation of people with mental health problems. They have done much to promote user/survivor-run and self-help alternatives to traditional mental health services (e.g. Chamberlin 1977, Lindow 1994), as well as working to improve the situation of people within mainstream services.

Once again, it is important to stress that there can be no prescriptions for the 'right' way for people to accommodate mental health problems into their lives. People differ on a multitude of dimensions: history, situation, life experiences, politics, philosophy, culture, ambitions, and aspirations. All of these factors will contribute to the ways in which they choose to accommodate their mental health problems. It is not the role of the practitioner to tell people what is best, but they can help them to explore different possibilities and work out, for themselves, an approach that makes sense to them.

PROMOTING PERSONAL ADJUSTMENT AND PSYCHOLOGICAL ADAPTATION

People can gain the support they need to accommodate what has happened to them from a variety of sources: friends, family, and, most especially, others who have experienced mental health problems. Mental health workers can, however, be an important source of help in what can be a time-consuming process. In this and subsequent chapters, a number of different ways of coping, managing and moving beyond problems are described. Although they are listed separately, in reality they overlap and are interlinked; they do not follow in any set order, as different people may prefer to start in different places. Some of the strategies and approaches outlined will be relevant to some people and not others. A person may wish to grapple with different issues at different times and may return to the same issue on a number of occasions. If the mental health workers are to assist in this process, they must be able to respond flexibly to the person's wishes and preferences, and, most importantly, recognise that most people are not starting from 'square one'. They are building on the wisdom they have already accumulated, the lessons they have already learned, and the competencies and coping skills that they have already developed.

Grieving that which has been lost

People need space and time to grieve, and to tell their life stories (over and over again if necessary, as new issues, meaning and understanding can emerge with each telling). In reclaiming a sense of identity and value in the present, it is often necessary for a person to talk of identities and valued roles of the past, and to express at least some of the anger, fear, despair, resentment or shame that they may feel over what has happened.

Practitioners may be uncomfortable with displays of emotion. On the one hand, it is not easy to witness the pain and grief of another person, especially if you cannot alleviate that pain and feel powerless to change the circumstances that produced it. It is therefore tempting to avoid touching upon those areas of a person's life that are likely to trigger such an emotional response. On the other hand, anger, fear and despair on the part of someone who is experiencing mental health problems are too often interpreted as symptoms that must be treated or avoided, rather than as an ordinary and understandable response to devastating events. When people become emotional, it is too easy to conclude that they cannot cope with the stress of thinking about what has happened. There is a delicate balance to be struck between helping people to express their feelings and forcing them to address issues that they do not yet have the personal resources to deal with. However, it is a grave error to prevent or pathologise all expressions of emotion. If people are to regain confidence in themselves, they need to regain confidence in their feelings – to understand that many of their emotions are ordinary and understandable responses. As Deegan (1993) put it, 'by extinguishing someone's anger . . . we run the risk of breaking their spirit and wounding their dignity'.

The process of grieving what has been lost may be slow, and the mental health worker must be able to cope with the person's distress. It is difficult to live with mental health problems and there may be little we can do to change the realities of the situation, but we can share the person's burden by understanding, empathising with, and accepting their distress. We can help that person to see that he/she is not alone.

Sometimes the anger may be directed at the mental health worker and the advantages that they have. Most practitioners may not feel privileged, but, in comparison with many of those with whom they work, they are very fortunate. Often it can be helpful for a person to meet others who are in a similar position, or people who have 'been there'. This may be achieved either by meeting them in person or through their writing; both can enable a person to see that there is a way of surviving the pain and moving forward (Kirkpatrick et al 2001).

For some people, the grieving process includes coming to terms with having done things that they find unacceptable. For example, one devout Catholic woman with whom we worked was mortified that, when 'high', she had run up and down the street and into the church with no clothes on. She was appalled at the thought of having to face her neighbours, and the priest, after having done this. Accepting that you have done things that you deem wrong is a challenge which people accommodate in different ways. For example, some find solace in religion, and others gain comfort from making amends, apologising or planning ways in which they can avoid doing similar things in the future. Others find the idea of illness, or extreme stress and adversity, a useful way of understanding why they behaved as they did. Everyone, at some time in life, does things that are regrettable, and everyone has had to find some way of forgiving himself/herself.

Information: challenging the myths

Many of the popular myths and misconceptions that surround mental health problems are inevitably shared by those who experience them, and are regularly reinforced in the popular media. These make the experience even more frightening. Many of those who deny that they have mental health problems do so in order to reject the images of themselves as dangerous and incompetent. Information is necessary to dispel the myths, and every practitioner should have, at his/her fingertips, facts and figures with which they can challenge the media barrage (Harding & Zahniser 1994), e.g.:

◆ 'People with mental health problems are dangerous.' In 1995, 522 people were convicted of homicide but only 60 of these were people who have a diagnosis of mental health problems. People who are drunk are far more likely to kill someone than people who have mental health problems. The vast majority of people with mental health problems never harm anyone.

◆ 'I will be stuck in this place forever.' Last year, half of the people who were living in this hostel moved on.

◆ 'I will never have a place of my own.' Over 99% of people who have longer term mental health problems live outside hospital: some live in hostels or with their families, but 75% have a place of their own.

◆ 'If I have children, they will get mental health problems like me.' Of children who have a parent with serious mental health problems, 90% do not develop mental health difficulties themselves. And are mental health problems really the 'end of the world'?

◆ 'I'll never get a job.' Nationally, about 18% of people with more serious mental health problems are in work, but research shows that, with the proper help, as many as 60% of people who have such difficulties can work successfully in real jobs (Bond et al 1997, 2001, Crowther et al 2001).

◆ 'People with mental health problems can never amount to very much – never do anything important.' There are many who have achieved great things, e.g. Van Gogh, Einstein, James Joyce, and Churchill all had mental health problems.

Individual stories of the 'I knew a woman who . . .' variety can also be valuable, but the personal accounts of people who have succeeded in rebuilding their lives can be even more powerful. There are a number of anthologies in which these can be found (see, for example, Spaniol & Koehler 1994, Read & Reynolds 1996), as well as papers in journals such as *Schizophrenia Bulletin* (see, for example, Leete 1988b, 1989). However, it is important to guard against making an individual feel a greater failure because he/she has 'failed' where others have succeeded. It may be helpful to acknowledge that things can be more difficult for people who have mental health problems, not only because of the difficulties themselves, but also because of the prejudice and discrimination that exist. Things can be difficult but are not impossible with the right kind of help and support.

Sometimes people with mental health problems are not willing to articulate their beliefs about madness because they are too frightening to contemplate. It may therefore be helpful for the mental health worker to be more proactive in articulating and refuting common preconceptions. There is nothing to be gained, however, from entering into a protracted battle with people who are adamant that they do not have mental health problems: acceptance of mental health difficulties is not a prerequisite for recovery. It is preferable to focus on helping people to do the things they want to do, or address the practical problems they experience (e.g. unemployment, lack of money, few friends), as they perceive them.

Understanding what has happened

When mental health workers talk about helping people to understand their problems, this is often taken to mean giving them technical descriptions of the faulty action of neurotransmitters and the symptoms that are thought to result from this. However, a cursory glance at the professional literature indicates that practitioners find it very difficult to agree on the most appropriate explanatory models. Organic, social, political, psychological, psychoanalytic and systemic theories continue to vie for supremacy, and it is increasingly accepted that a variety of social, environmental, biological and psychological processes may be involved.

Like the professionals, people who experience mental health problems adopt a range of different explanatory models to understand the problems that they experience. Jacobson (1993) analysed the personal narratives of 30 people who had themselves faced the challenge of recovery; she identified six different approaches that people had employed. Each implied a different model of understanding of what had happened, and different sources of help. However, she found commonalities in people's understanding of recovery regardless of which of the six paths were taken:

◆ Biological Model. In line with a biomedical model, some people emphasise the importance of understanding the disease and its treatment. They accept help in order to control their symptoms, and consider the major challenge to involve integrating their illness into their concept of self: 'to know yourself, to know your illness, and to know the difference between the two' (Anon 1995).

◆ Abuse or Trauma Model (e.g. Schmook 1994, Bova 1995). Other people see their difficulties as arising from the pain of severe trauma, which causes them to lose their sense of self and to behave in ways which others define as deviant. When this deviance brought them into the mental health system, this became a further source of abuse or trauma. Recovery involves taking back control over their life by changing internal and external conditions.

◆ Biological and Environmental Model (e.g. Frese 1997). Some people explain their difficulties as an innate biological vulnerability that becomes a full-blown mental illness in stressful conditions (this approach is similar to the stress-vulnerability model described by Zubin & Spring 1977). Recovery involves managing one's symptoms, reducing exposure to stressful situations, setting goals, and finding strategies for managing everyday life.

◆ Spiritual or Philosophical Model (e.g. Alexander 1994). Some people explain their problems in terms of a spiritual or philosophical crisis that destroys the spirit and then recreates a new 'truth'. What others see does not represent the individual's own experience, so standard interventions are unhelpful. The greatest source of help is connection with some source of enlightenment, e.g. Buddhism, the Bible, the Koran, treatises of philosophy or physics, etc.

◆ Political Model (Curtis et al 2000). For some people, mental illness does not exist, and the mental health system itself is viewed as the problem. It is felt to deprive marginalised individuals of their human and civil rights to ensure that they can be no threat. Recovery involves politicisation, i.e. finding a framework that enables them to reject the identity of 'mental patient' and place their experiences in a broader context of power and powerlessness. Anger that may previously have been turned inwards can then be transformed into political action designed to change the system. The individual may join with other 'survivors' to effect social change.

◆ Spirit-breaking Model (e.g. Deegan 1993, 1996). For others, the major problems are a consequence of the dehumanising effect of long-term contact with the mental health system. The hopelessness of figures of power within the system is spirit-breaking. Recovery begins when a spark of hope and courage is ignited and then maintained by the support of family, friends, peers and professionals.

What is clear is that a recovery vision does not require a person to adopt any particular model or understanding of his/her difficulties. Practitioners should not see their role as persuading the person of the 'correct' way to understand their situation. Veracity is not the key issue as far as recovery is concerned. The critical thing is that the person finds a way of understanding what has happened that satisfies two criteria: it must both *make sense to him/her and offer the possibility of actively moving forward and rebuilding his/her life.*

For the practitioner, the first step must be to listen to the person's account of his/her life and problems and pay attention to the types of explanation already being used. Perhaps family and relationship problems are emphasised, in which case social models and the impact of stressors may make most sense to the client. If the individual talks about how his/her mother or father had similar problems, then that person will be more inclined to accept some form of genetic vulnerability explanation. If he/she sees the world in religious or spiritual terms, then he/she is likely to seek an explanation for the problems within that framework.

Sometimes a person may be adopting a number of different frameworks at different levels or to explain different problems. For example, they may see themselves as having an illness that has been made worse by the dehumanising effect of the mental health system. Other people may be confused, or unsure, about how to understand their difficulties. If so, the practitioner might usefully describe a range of different ways in which people have sought understanding (see, for example, Jacobson 1993, above or Coleman & Smith 1997a,b) and explore which makes most sense to the person.

The explanatory framework that a person uses does not automatically imply a given set of interventions. One gentleman with whom we worked attributed his difficulties to abuse within his family, but considered that these had resulted in damage to his thinking process, for which he required the help of drugs. Another, whose cognitive problems made it difficult for him to pray, believed this to be the work of the devil, but found medication helpful, not in curing his problems, but in countering the devil's influence.

The most important feature of the explanatory framework is the extent to which it offers hope for the future and the possibility of being an active agent. Some interpretations deny this possibility, leading people to believe that there is nothing that they, themselves, can do. They may believe that all is hopeless (for example, 'I have committed such a terrible sin that I must be punished – there is no redemption', 'It's in my blood/genes' so that is that.'), or that they must simply wait for someone else to do something or for something else to happen (e.g. wait for the drugs to work, or for their mother to behave differently, or for the system to change). All of these are powerless positions that deny agency.

If the person's chosen interpretation does not allow them room for manoeuvre, then instead of trying to replace the framework with another, it is usually more sensible for the mental health worker to seek alternatives *within* the person's chosen framework. For example, if a person believes his/her problems to be inherited, he/she may see this as meaning that his/her life is entirely predetermined and there is nothing that can be done. This type of construction severely limits the possibilities and is likely to result in hopelessness and despair. The practitioner could encourage that person to explore other possibilities supported by genetic evidence. Even if both parents have a diagnosis of schizophrenia there is only a 46% chance of their child developing schizophrenia. This indicates how the action of genes can be modified by social, experiential and environmental factors. Perhaps the client could entertain a 'stress-vulnerability' model in which his/her genes leave him/her vulnerable to problems, but it is various stressors that trigger episodes of illness. This would allow that person to begin to identify stressful situations, think about ways of avoiding them, and deal differently with the stresses and strains of everyday life (see Chapter 8).

However, it is not simply an understanding of symptoms that people with mental health problems seek. Many people do not think too deeply about the meaning of life until something happens that shakes them to the core: the death of a long-term partner, being made redundant, retirement, or children leaving home can all trigger a major re-evaluation. Serious mental health problems can have a similar impact, prompting people to ask questions like 'Why me?', 'What's the point in life?' and 'Why should I carry on?'. When people's confidence has been eroded it is easy for them to see little point, believing that their life is over. But there are other ways of understanding the meaning of life.

Over the centuries, people have adopted a range of religious and spiritual beliefs in which they find hope for the future. Others may find meaning in humanistic – or a range of non-religious political – frameworks, which hold that every human life is valuable and that 'perfection' is not a desirable or ethical goal. Perhaps a person may find meaning in the creative power of suffering – much great art and literature derives not from happiness but from adversity – or in the positive contribution that people with mental health problems can make to humanity in terms of increased understanding and sensitivity. Perhaps there may be political beliefs relating to the celebration of social diversity and the importance of inclusion, or scientific beliefs about the importance of diversity in the gene pool enabling the human race to survive different threats. Some genetic 'clouds' may have silver linings (in the same way that sickle cell is protective against malaria). The possibilities are manifold.

Many workers may be uncomfortable with such philosophical questions, but these may be important in rekindling the meaning, purpose and hope necessary for recovery. Many practitioners will have strongly held beliefs in these areas, and it is important that these are not used prescriptively. The aim is to help the person explore what makes sense for him/her. Helping people to access the ways in which others have addressed challenges they have faced can be helpful. Within the mental health field, texts like *From the Ashes of Experience* (Barker et al 1999) might be useful, but important lessons can also be learned from people who have faced other types of adversity. Examples include Bauby's account of his persistent vegetative state in *The Butterfly and the Diving Bell* (1998) (which he laboriously dictated by means of the slight remaining movement in one eye lid), Ruth Picardie's account of terminal cancer in *Before I Say Goodbye* (1998), and Brian Keenan's account of his years as a hostage in the Lebanon in *An Evil Cradling* (1993).

REBUILDING A SENSE OF SELF: REDISCOVERING MEANING AND PURPOSE

The experience of mental health problems can severely threaten a person's sense of self; too many people are reduced to little more than their 'illness' and being a 'mental patient'. The ways in which this occurs are described by many people who have experienced mental health problems (see, for example, Deegan 1988, 1993, Leete 1988a). As Davidson & Strauss (1992) have argued, 'the process of rediscovering and reconstructing an enduring sense of the self as an active and responsible agent provides an important, and perhaps crucial, source of growth in the recovery process'. On the basis of interviews with 66 people who had experienced serious and prolonged mental health difficulties, these authors identified four basic aspects of the reconstruction of self:

◆ discovering the possibility a more active sense of self
◆ taking stock of the strengths and weaknesses of this self and assessing the possibilities for change

◆ putting into action some aspects of that self in order to discover your capabilities

◆ using the enhanced sense of self to cope with the symptoms, discrimination and prejudice experienced.

Mental health workers may be able to help a person to rediscover and rebuild a sense of self in a number of ways. Believing in that person's possibilities is crucial. It is difficult to develop a sense of yourself unless others believe in you, and such belief is lacking in a world which devalues and excludes people with mental health problems. The practitioner may therefore have an important role in holding on to that belief and hope. As Betty (cited in Davidson & Strauss, 1992) describes:

> ...it may have been because [my nurse] really seemed to pay a lot of particular attention to me...I started waking up and I started knowing that there were possibilities for life outside that room and things really started opening up for me....she knew I had potential and talent and all this and that I could get better, and I knew it too.

Our sense of self is often built on an understanding of our history. We understand ourselves in the present with reference to how we came to be here. Our histories are not fixed and given entities. Each of us attaches different meaning to those places we have visited, to those things that have happened to us and to those things we have done. The significance and meaning we attach to events can change, and these changes can determine the way in which we see ourselves in the present. The way we tell our story influences how we see ourselves and our sense of agency.

Storytelling – experimenting with different ways of understanding where we have been in order to see where we can go – can be important. This story is not the same as the psychiatric history that is inevitably present in a person's file. A psychiatric history is the story of illness. In rebuilding a sense of self, the important story is a personal story of life that enables someone to move beyond what has happened. Some people may prefer to recount these stories verbally, while others may prefer to write them down. Sometimes it is helpful for practitioner and client to work out the story together and then write it down so that the person has something tangible to hold on to.

It is important that in telling this story a person moves beyond a catalogue of events (born in London, went to St George's school, etc.) to thinking about what these things meant for him/her – at the time and with the benefit of hindsight. A number of recovery texts and workbooks have suggested headings that the person might use in order to think about their story (see, for example, Coleman & Smith 1997a,b, Coleman 1999). As well as details of significant events (birth, school, marriage, hospitalisation) these include formative experiences in childhood, adolescence and adulthood, those things that the person sees as having been important in shaping his/her life. It is helpful to discover why these things might have been so important. As well as thinking about problems and traumas, people should be encouraged to think about things they have valued, about achievements and about those things of which they are proud.

There are number of people who find other forms of writing helpful in the process of understanding themselves and making sense of their situations. Some find it useful to write diaries. Others find meaning through poetry and songwriting, and come together to do this in music projects (such as Sound Minds in Wandsworth) or organisations like Survivors' Poetry.

People need to think about where they have been. They also need to consider where they are now and where they are going. To identify personal, social and material assets, the problems of which they are often so painfully aware, and the possibilities for the future (Davidson & Strauss 1992). People may need to try out a multitude of different ways of seeing themselves and the future, 'trying on' a number of different identities to see which suit them. It is important that practitioners facilitate this exploration rather than sticking with the first possibility that emerges. For example, one young man we worked with initially saw his future as being 'one of the lads'. He wanted to be one of the local gang – 'a lager lout'. With support, he started to go to football matches again, and to 'hang out' in a local pub he had enjoyed. However, he found that this did not offer what he had hoped, and decided instead that he needed to improve his education. He tried various courses but completed none before deciding that he was too old for education and needed a job, so we began working on this. Initially he worked in a voluntary capacity before going to the local job centre and exploring the possibility of vocational training courses and paid work.

It can be very frustrating if people frequently change their mind about what they want to do ('I went to all that trouble to help him get into that college course, and he just gave it up.'). It is easy to conclude that a person 'lacks motivation' or 'is unable to make up his mind' and be reluctant to help him/her try other things. It is important to remember, however, that most of us had to try out many different possibilities and ways of being before we found out who we wanted to be and what we wanted to do, and in the future we may well decide again to re-evaluate what we are doing and even change course. If we are to facilitate someone's recovery we must help him/her in these explorations. It may also be helpful to support that person in reflecting on what he/she has done in order to inform future decisions.

As the example of the 'lager lout' illustrates, in developing the sense of an active self, it is necessary to put that self into action. If the person doubts his/her abilities, then the initial steps may need to be small so that the person can see that it is possible to achieve something. The person may need a great deal of help if he/she is to risk 'having a go'. This help may need to be low key and unobtrusive if pride and confidence are not to be further eroded. It is difficult for anyone to accept help with things that most people find easy or that we used to be able to do unaided. As well as providing support to access opportunities, it may be necessary for the practitioner to help someone work out how to cope with ongoing symptoms and problems. It is to ways in which mental health workers can enable people to put their 'self' into action that we now turn.

The acceptance of what has happened and the rebuilding of a sense of self do not occur in a vacuum.

8

Facilitating personal adaptation: taking back control

An essential element of rebuilding a meaningful and valuable life with mental health problems involves taking back control. Recovery means 'being in the driving seat' (Deegan 1989, Glover 2001). This involves taking control of cognitive and emotional difficulties as well as making decisions for yourself about the way in which you live your life.

> To me, recovery means I try to stay in the driver's seat of my life. I don't let my illness run me. Over the years I have worked hard to become an expert in my own self-care. For me, being in recovery means I don't just take medications. Just taking medications is a passive stance. Rather I use medications as part of my recovery process. In the same way, I don't just go into hospital. Just 'going into hospital' is a passive stance. Rather, I use the hospital when I need to. (Deegan 1989)

In order to make decisions for ourselves, we first need to believe that this is possible, to understand that we are the experts on our own mental health problems. It is only the person himself/herself who can really know the effectiveness of different medications or coping strategies, what the side-effects feel like, and how they respond to difficult situations. However, mental health workers can have an important influence – for good or ill. Relationships with mental health workers can form a basis for developing self-belief and support the person in taking risks and making discoveries. But, if people are to take back control, then practitioners must recognise people's existing skills and coping strategies and help them to develop these to manage their own difficulties.

Traditionally, people have looked to professionals to provide answers, and the professions have developed on the basis of their supposedly unique expertise and exclusive knowledge. If we are to respect the expertise of personal experience, however, then mental health workers must use their expertise in a different way. Rather than making decisions for people, professional, must put our knowledge at the disposal of the people with whom we work so that they can make decisions for themselves. Chapter 12 discusses the issues involved in changing the balance of power within the mental health services. This chapter explores the strategies that people with mental health problems have found helpful in minimising and coping with their cognitive and emotional difficulties, in managing crises and relapses, and in maintaining helpful relationships with families and friends. Our aim here is not to provide a detailed account of all the different interventions and approaches; these can be found elsewhere (c.f. Birchwood & Tarrier 1992, Brooker & Repper 1998). Instead, we offer an overview of some of the different approaches that can be used to help people take back control.

MINIMISING SYMPTOMS

There is no intervention that can 'cure' mental health problems in the sense that, for example, antibiotics can eliminate some bacterial infections, but there are many forms of help that can alleviate or control unpleasant and intrusive symptoms. Over the past decade there have been great advances in psychological and social strategies to help people with mental health problems. Yet, since the discovery of the effect of phenothiazines on symptoms of schizophrenia (over 50 years ago), drugs remain the most common form of help offered. There are many people who find that some drugs can be helpful in minimising the distressing symptoms that they experience. However, it remains the case that too many people who come into contact with mental health services are offered little other than medication. There may be a number of reasons for this.

First, it is doctors – whether they be general practitioners or psychiatrists – who are generally the first port of call for people with mental health problems. Many psychiatrists would now adopt a 'bio-psycho-social' approach and see the importance of a range of different interventions outside the pharmacological domain. However, their primary competencies and models remain largely 'organic'. As Thomas (1997), himself a psychiatrist, writes:

> What exactly do psychiatrists mean when they use the word [schizophrenia]? The best way to answer this question is to describe it in terms of epidemiology, genetics, biochemistry, neurodevelopment and cognition. These theories provide much of the scientific basis underlying modern approaches to treatment and therapy.

Second, people with serious mental health problems have traditionally been considered 'unsuitable' for 'talking therapies'. This may be because of their supposed 'lack of contact with reality' or 'lack of insight' (Perkins &

Repper 1996), or because of their 'poor social skills' whereby they may find eye contact difficult, be slow to answer, or need help to understand what is meant by the questions (Frese 1997). Alternatively, it may be assumed that they lack the 'ego-strength' necessary for traditional insight-orientated therapies (Bachrach 1982).

Whilst these misinformed presumptions persist in some areas, it is increasingly considered appropriate to offer both medication and psychological interventions to minimise, or allow the client to cope with, cognitive and emotional difficulties. However, there remains a shortage of practitioners skilled in psychological therapies, and those who are available have tended to work with people who are less disabled by their mental health problems. For example, most in-patients do not have access to clinical psychologists and psychotherapists, who continue to spend the vast majority of their time in out-patient clinics.

MEDICATION

A range of different drugs are available for people who experience mental health problems. It is widely recognised that most of these have both positive and negative effects, and that individuals differ in their responses. As the *British National Formulary* (cited in Pratt 1998) states, 'The difference between the various anti-psychotics is less important than the variability in patient response to the individual drug.' Some people have argued that medication will 'provide the necessary foundation for recovery' (Francell 2002), but many others have focused on the debilitating side-effects that it can have. This range of opinion and response is reflected in the accounts of people with experience of taking these drugs:

> *Without major tranquillisers myself and my family feel I may not have survived, as hyperactivity and starvation led to rapid weight loss as well as psychological symptoms.*

> *The drugs block out most of the damaging voices and delusions and keep my mood stable.*

> *Injections seem to dampen down the voices. They decrease the voices but not altogether, and the side effects are unpleasant.*

> *They do not cure the cause of conditions; they have the side effects of making you unnaturally doped, enormously fat.*

> *With major tranquillisers, I feel as if I'm in a trance. I don't feel like myself.* (all cited in British Psychological Society 2000)

All drug treatments must be considered in the context of the extent to which facilitate people doing the things they want to do. To this extent a balance must be achieved between the beneficial effects and the problems associated with treatment – and this balance will be different for every individual. For one person, the voices may be so intolerable that he/she is willing to put up with side-effects. For another, the side-effects may be so intolerable that he/she would rather put up with the symptoms. Different people will have different opinions about the balance between symptom relief and side-effects, and it is important to respect these opinions. The nature and severity of side-effects will have different significance for different people: sexual dysfunction may be distressing for most people, but for some it will be less problematic than for others; weight gain may be more of a deterrent to taking medication for some people than for others. We cannot make assumptions about any of these things, so every individual needs to be given full and honest information and the opportunity to try different drugs, doses and combinations.

Often, the issue that is of concern to people is not one of medication *per se*, but one of control – or, rather, lack of control. Clearly, for medication to be tailored to the needs and lifestyle of an individual, that person must play an active part in decisions about which drug is taken, not to mention how much, when and in what form. In order to make such decisions, information, negotiation, choice and experimentation are important. These depend on the willingness of the prescriber to listen to, and heed, the client's opinions. All too often, drugs are prescribed with little discussion about effects, side-effects and alternatives (Sandford 1994), and people are encouraged to believe that they must passively accept the 'doctor's orders'. As Francell (2002), who himself has a diagnosis of bipolar disorder, observes:

> *Many consumers still think of psychiatrists as glorified gurus of medication, so there is no need to learn anything or ask questions. All one has to do is 'pop pills' and see the 'shrink' every so often. The term for this kind of thinking is called passive recipiency, and it can stifle recovery. In my experience, recovery began when I got off the bench and became an active player in the treatment game. Often, one needs guidance and patience to make the shift from spectator to player.*

One consequence of seeing yourself as a 'spectator' is that there is an assumption that you *have* to take what is offered or receive no help at all. Many people feel pressured into taking medication (Luckstead & Coursey 1995), most commonly by verbal persuasion but also by the threat posed by the very existence of mental health legislation (Wallcraft 2002). The power and status of mental health professionals mean that many people will unquestioningly accept their prescriptions, and, if they do not, then other sanctions can be invoked. These may take the form of complete withdrawal of assistance ('You can only stay here if you take the medication.') or legal compulsion.

If a person refuses to take medication, then he/she is likely to be deemed 'non-compliant'. Such 'non-compliance' has been viewed as the cause of most relapses, readmissions, and high-profile 'failures of community care'. It has been claimed that 'non-compliance' is associated with 43% of admissions (Kent & Yellowlees 1994) and an estimated cost of around £100 million per year (Davis & Drummond 1990). The typical argument is summarised by Kemp et al (1996):

> *Given the established efficacy of neuroleptic drugs in psychotic disorders, and the potentially devastating consequences of relapse, non-compliance is one of the major preventable causes of psychiatric morbidity and a research priority for the NHS.*

Concerns about 'non-compliance' have resulted in the development of interventions to reduce it. 'Compliance therapy' is one approach that has been developed to increase 'insight' and 'compliance with medication'. It involves a three-stage process:

> *1. Elicit patient's stance towards treatment (including: review history, formulate stance towards treatment, link medication cessation and relapse, meet denial with gentle enquiry, acknowledge negative treatment experiences, suggest advantage of patient's involvement in own treatment).*
> *2. Explore ambivalence to treatment (including: predict common misgivings about treatment, correct misperceptions, guide considerations of benefits and drawbacks of treatment, use metaphors (e.g. medication as a protective layer), highlight indirect benefits of treatment, cautiously explore delusional resistance to treatment).*
> *3. Working towards treatment maintenance (including: encourage self-efficacy, medication as a positive strategy to enhance quality of life, illness as the hand of cards life has dealt you, emphasise prevalence and well known sufferers, analogy to physical illness needing long term treatment, predict consequences of stopping treatment, identify prodromal symptoms, value of staying well, medication as insurance policy to stay well).* (Kemp et al 1997)

Although the authors emphasise the importance of working on an individualised basis, and aiming for 'self-efficacy', this approach is not concerned with giving information so that the person can make an informed choice. Rather, it constitutes a programme designed to persuade people to understand and accept the clinician's point of view (gain insight) and take their pills. Such an approach runs counter to national policy directives requiring that services be tailored to the wishes and priorities of those who use them (Department of Health 1999, 2000a). Yet increasing numbers of mental health workers are receiving compliance-therapy training.

Perhaps the most worrying aspect of 'compliance therapy' is the assumption that 'non-compliance' is irrational, i.e. a function of the 'lack of insight' that is supposedly inherent in some mental health problems. But Diamond (1983), himself a psychiatrist, warns, 'Clinicians may sometimes be too quick to blame non-compliance rather than non-effectiveness when drugs do not help a psychiatric patient.' It should be noted that people who do not have mental health problems are equally likely to be 'non-compliant' with medication: around 50% of patients do not take medication for physical ailments in accordance with instructions (Sackett 1976). Such 'non-compliance' is often a rational act (Perkins & Repper 1998) and may arise for a number of reasons (outlined below):

◆ the perceived ineffectiveness of the drug (Ruscher et al 1997)
◆ the complexity of the drug regime (Blackwell 1972, Eisen & Miller 1990)
◆ the presence of unpleasant side-effects (Blackwell 1972, Fleischtaker et al 1994)
◆ a belief that medication is not necessary, (Donovan & Blake 1992)
◆ a poor relationship with the prescriber, leading to a lack of trust in their prescriptions (Blackwell 1972, Garrity 1981, Frank et al 1995)
◆ lack of choice and involvement in the prescribing of medication (Conrad 1985).

Rather than pathologising individuals for not taking medication we must explore the complex issues involved:

◆ Sometimes a person may want to take medication but finds difficulties in doing so. If the problem lies in remembering to take it, then simple reminders – a note on the fridge door or the bathroom cupboard – may help. If he/she has difficulty collecting the prescription, then maybe the doctor could send it to the person's home, or someone could collect it on his/her behalf.

◆ Sometimes, on the basis of past experience, the person may prefer a different type or dosage of medication; such personal experience should be heeded.

◆ Sometimes the person is experiencing distressing side-effects. These should be taken seriously and ways of alleviating them addressed. Perhaps a reduction in dosage, or a change of medication, may help. Alternatively, non-pharmacological treatments may be preferable.

Information is always necessary to enable people to make informed choices. Information about side-effects does not necessarily mean that a person will be unwilling to take the drug: knowing about possible effects can make these less frightening if they occur. However, mental health workers cannot assume that people will always draw the same conclusions from the information with which they are provided. Nor can we, as practitioners, assume that we have a monopoly on relevant information. People with mental health problems know what taking different types of medication feels like – information that mental health workers often lack and that cannot be readily acquired from textbooks. We have much to learn from those who have first-hand experience.

Coping with specific symptoms

If people are to take back control of their lives, they need to be able to manage the cognitive and emotional difficulties that have got in the way. A 'stress-vulnerability' model (Zubin & Spring 1977) may be helpful in doing this. This approach proposes that people may be vulnerable to mental health problems as a result of a number of factors outwith their control (including genetic influences, adversity, trauma and poor parenting). But it is everyday stressors and life events that trigger problematic symptoms – and people can gain control over these. People can identify the stressor that causes them problems and work out ways of dealing with them. As Esso Leete (1989) says:

> . . . *stress does play an enormous part in my illness [schizophrenia]. There are enormous pressures that come with any new experience and environment, and any change, positive or negative, is extremely difficult. What ever I can do to decrease or avoid high stress environments is helpful in controlling my symptoms. In general terms all of my coping strategies consist of four steps: (1) recognizing when I am feeling stressed, which is harder than it may sound; (2) identifying the stressor; (3) remembering from past experience what action helped in the same situation or a similar one; and (4) taking that action as quickly as possible after I have identified the source of stress.* (Leete 1989)

Leete (1989) goes on to enumerate the coping strategies that she has developed to deal with the specific problems that she experiences.

◆ She copes with a chaotic inner existence by adopting a highly structured daily schedule, carefully planned use of time, 'compulsive organisation', limited leisure – unstructured time.

◆ She finds work therapeutic as it is a structured activity, something to look forward to, a skill to learn and improve. It gives a sense of productivity, increased confidence, a sense of worth that replaces usual feelings of incompetence, decreases stigma, and contributes to acceptance in the community.

◆ She copes with difficulties in filtering or screening out irrelevant stimuli by reducing distractions as much as possible.

◆ She copes with contradictory feelings of loneliness and isolation, and fear of close friendships, by socializing with people who share her interests.

◆ She finds numerous acquaintances useful but accepts her reduced capacity for close friendships.

◆ She finds peer-run support groups useful as a means of both accepting and dealing with mental illness.

◆ She copes with difficulty in making eye contact by looking up intermittently in conversations – but just past the other person.

◆ She withdraws to another room to be alone for a while if overwhelmed in a social situation.

◆ She tries to keep in touch with feelings and attend to difficulties immediately.

◆ She anticipates paranoid feelings and takes preventive action, e.g. instead of worrying about the police surprising her, she always sits facing the door with her back to the wall.

◆ She tests reality with someone she trusts: if their perceptions are different from hers, she may want to change her response and go along with more conventional ways of thinking rather than incorporating more external information into her delusional system.

◆ She copes with impaired concentration and memory by making lists, concentrates intensely for short periods of time, takes extra time, and tries to be persistent.

◆ She breaks tasks down into small steps, takes one at a time, and recognises the achievement of small goals because this builds her confidence about doing other things.

◆ She finds ambiguity, complexity and vagueness difficult so asks others to communicate in a clear, specific and simple way.

◆ She may need extra time in conversations, to give her time to think before responding.

◆ She copes with high levels of ambivalence by asking for extra time to make decisions.

◆ She remains aware of her need to fit in: she tries not to talk to herself or to her voices in the presence of others, and does whatever makes her feel better in a way that does not look bizarre. For example, if she needs to rock, she sits in a rocking chair, hammock or swing or if she needs to pace, she goes for a walk.

A problem-solving framework

Leete has clearly identified the situations that present most difficulty for her, has worked out the strategies that are most effective in those situations, and deliberately uses these strategies to avoid undue stress or worsening symptoms. Mental health workers can help people to develop their own ways of coping through the sort of problem-solving process that Leete (1989) describes. This involves determining the most difficult problem or situation that a person faces and negotiating a strategy for coping with that situation. A problem-solving framework (Perkins & Repper 1996, Kingdon 1998) can be useful in addressing ordinary everyday problems (such as relationship difficulties or problems with money), but it can also be useful in addressing specific cognitive and emotional difficulties (such as 'voices' or unusual beliefs interfering with the things a person wants to do, or difficulties in going outside the house) .

Identifying the specific problem

Sometimes people describe their difficulties in specific terms ('I get frightened waiting for my benefits because the other people in the queue talk about me.') but more usually we think about them in a broad, general way ('No one likes me.', 'I can't get up in the mornings.'). Before solutions can be sought, it is necessary for the person to explore exactly what the difficulties are: 'I find it hard to go to sleep at night. I am often awake until 3 am because the neighbours make so much noise and then I am exhausted when it is time to get up.' Often it is helpful to think back to the last time the problem occurred and to describe the events leading up to it (Did you have problems getting up this morning? Think back to the evening before. What time did you go to bed? Did you go to sleep? What stopped you sleeping?' etc.). People often feel very alone with their problems; it can be reassuring to meet, or read about, others who have similar difficulties and who can also provide helpful tips about ways of dealing with such problems.

Sometimes people have a number of difficulties and need to prioritise which ones they want to address first. Some might prefer to start with those which are the most distressing or disabling, but others might find these too daunting and prefer to try something more manageable first. For example, one man's 'voices' prevented him from going out, but they also stopped him reading the newspaper. The problems with going out were more of a barrier to him doing the things he wanted to do, but he could not contemplate working on this straightaway. Therefore he worked on being able to read the paper; the strategies he discovered for doing this were helpful when he later tackled his difficulties in going out.

Throughout, it is important to remember that people must define the things that are difficult for them. A mental health worker may, for example, see 'voices' as, by definition, problematic, whereas the person him/herself finds them companionable and comforting and no barrier to doing the things he/she wants to do. Equally, being able to cook may not present a difficulty. How many of us rely on snacks, ready meals and take-aways? Problems are specific to the person who experiences them – what *they* find distressing and what *they* want to achieve.

Identifying possible courses of action

In seeking solutions to a problem, creativity is of the essence. The first step is to think about all the possible ways of dealing with it. Some of these will involve ways of eliminating the difficulty (e.g. reducing the fear of going out alone) while others may involve ways of stopping the problem interfering so much with the person's life (e.g. ways of finding other people to accompany the person when he/she goes out). In both cases, the quest for ways of dealing with difficulties is not simply a matter of the mental health worker prescribing courses of action. If the person is to grow and develop, he/she must be an active participant in the process. People will often have developed a number of solutions themselves; these provide a useful starting point. Many people can think of other possible strategies to try. In thinking about these, it can be helpful to ask them to think about what they might suggest to someone else who had similar difficulties. At other times people may need to do further research by asking others, especially others with similar difficulties, what they would suggest. It can be helpful to write down all the possible courses of action so that they are not forgotten.

People can discover all manner of different ways of coping. For example, we have known people who deal with their 'voices' by finding somewhere quiet to talk to them, going for a walk alone, talking to someone else, listening to music, reading, telling the 'voices' to go away, using earplugs, negotiating a time when they can talk to them, taking more medication, exercise, writing, and so on. One man found that if he spoke to his 'voices' in a foreign language then they thought they had got the wrong person and went away. Identifying the range of possible solutions can take time. However, it is not time wasted. The process of researching different ways of dealing with difficulties can be a source of hope in and of itself, providing evidence that the person is not as 'stuck' as he/she might have felt, and showing that there are ways forward; if one way does not work out, then another might.

Selecting a course of action

Having decided on the range of different ways of proceeding, the next step is to decide which strategy, or combination of strategies, to try first. What are the pros and cons of each? Which are feasible given the situation and the person's resources? Different solutions may be appropriate in different situations. For example, it may be possible to talk back to 'voices' when at home, but in the office it may be more difficult. Sometimes it may be necessary to decide on some immediate, 'stop-gap' measures while working on longer term resolutions. For example, a person might get a friend to collect his/her benefits while he/she works on being able to go out alone. Sometimes a hierarchical approach may be sensible: 'First I will try ignoring the "voices"; if they persist then I will go to a quiet place and reason with them, and if this doesn't work then I will listen to my personal stereo.' Each person needs to work out their own course of action but it can be helpful to have someone with whom to talk through the possibilities. This may be a mental health worker, but it can also be close friends, family members or others who have experienced similar difficulties.

Action

Once a person has selected a strategy, or series of strategies, the next step is to draw up a plan of action. Sometimes it is helpful to break the task down into smaller steps: 'In order to go out, first I will just walk to the gate, then I will try going a few steps along the street, then I will go to the corner shop...' Sometimes it is useful to recruit the help of someone else. Rehearsing what you are going to do in advance can make you feel more confident. Things can take time to work, and the person may become dispirited. Therefore it can be important to make sure that opportunities for support and encouragement are built in.

Reflection and review

An important part of taking back control involves learning from experience, reflecting on what has been achieved and reviewing possible ways forward. Progress is rarely smooth. There are likely to be setbacks as well as successes. If things have not worked out the first time, it is very easy for a person to feel disheartened and give up. So it can be helpful to have someone else around – whether this be a mental health worker or not – to provide support and encouragement and to think of different things to try. It is essential that the person providing this support is able to empathise with the individual sense of hopelessness (rather than simply telling him/her to 'pull himself/herself together'), while at the same time holding on to hope and believing that it is possible for that person to move forward. At such times, the list of possible courses of action developed earlier in the problem-solving process comes into its own. The person can go back and select different things they might try. However, it is equally important to recognize and celebrate successes along the way, however small these may seem.

This sort of 'problem-solving' approach is one that people use all the time – whether or not they have mental health difficulties. Many people find it helpful to have someone around to assist with the process. However, such assistance cannot be prescriptive. If the person is to take control of his/her own life, then the role of the helper is to share the journey and assist him/her to find his/her own solutions.

Sometimes, the process of exploration can reduce the problems themselves. People can re-evaluate their experiences, changing their beliefs about the world and their responses to it. At other times, the beliefs may continue, but their disruptive impact on the person's life can be reduced. For example, one person with whom we worked believed that he had AIDS. He had never tested positively for HIV, but had arrived at this conclusion following a prolonged bout of 'flu. He interpreted all aches and pains as confirmation of this belief, and felt sure that health professionals were deliberately withholding this information from him. His 'voices' made constant reference to his ill-health and accused him of spreading the infection. He was extremely distressed at the thought of infecting other people and was reluctant to go out in case he did so, and was preoccupied by his imminent death. In helping him to address these difficulties, the mental health worker assisted him in researching AIDS: it's symptoms, means of transmission, etc. As a result of this process, he recognized that he could go out without putting others at risk but should practice 'safe sex'. He also encountered people who did not see themselves as dying but as 'living with AIDS', and gradually recognized that, even if he was going to die, he could make the most of the time he had left and do the things he wanted to do. As a result, his preoccupation with death decreased. Although he continued to believe that he probably had AIDS, this belief ceased to control his whole life.

It is important to emphasise that the mental health worker did not take the approach of challenging this man's beliefs – 'reassuring' him that he did not have AIDS. Many people had taken this approach with the result that all his energies were devoted to proving that he did have it. Instead, the mental health worker joined him in an exploration of his beliefs, the bases for them, and the actions resulting from them. Sometimes such a 'testing' of our beliefs about ourselves and the world leads us to review and modify those beliefs. At other times, it reduces the distress associated with them and allows us to explore different – less restrictive – courses of action that we might take. On the basis of his research this man realised that he could go out and that practicing 'safe sex' was enough to prevent him infecting others. This type of approach is central to some of the cognitive-behavioural interventions that have been developed to help people who experience unusual beliefs and unshared perceptions (see Nelson 1997, Kingdon & Turkington 1994, Chadwick et al 1996).

In working with people whose beliefs are seen as 'delusional' it is essential that the mental health worker entertains the possibility that those beliefs could be true, even if he/she does not believe them to be so. Truth is not absolute. Different people see the world in different ways, many of which we may not share. However, if we cannot understand and accept a person's reality, then we cannot help them to explore it. Even if a person's thinking processes are deemed faulty, the content of their thoughts is important. Such content cannot be a direct consequence of neurotransmitter problems: it is not possible to believe that you are being influenced by the television in a society where televisions are unknown. The content of people's beliefs can reflect important facets of their experience. One woman we knew repeatedly told us 'I'm not a prostitute. They [the voices] say I'm a prostitute, but it's not true!'; she had been sexually abused as a child and told by her family that it was all her fault.

There are many different ways in which people can address the problems that they experience. Some people prefer to do this informally with friends, or in a self-help framework with others who experience similar difficulties. Such an approach can be seen in the 'self-management' programmes, developed by the Manic Depression Fellowship (www.mdf.org.uk), which are run by, and for, people who experience extreme mood swings. Some people find more formal therapy of assistance, while others prefer a more informal working relationship with a mental health worker. Others find self-help workbooks helpful. These include the *Victim to Victor* workbooks (Coleman & Smith 1997a,b) for people who hear 'voices' or harm themselves.

MANAGING CRISES AND RELAPSES

People with mental health problems can monitor their own 'ups and downs' (signs of impending difficulties) and often know when things are amiss long before this is evident to others. By doing this it is possible to manage problems before they become full-blown crises. Sometimes this can be achieved by the person themselves by, for example, cutting down on activities, drinking less, getting enough sleep, or sticking to a basic daily routine. It may involve enlisting the help of friends or family members. But there may be occasions on which the help of mental health professionals, adjustments in medication, or a period of respite care, is required.

The control of relapse is important. Not only does each relapse increase the possibility of further relapse (McGlashen 1988) and residual symptoms (Hogarty et al 1991), it also diminishes self-confidence and disrupts roles and relationships. Recovery may be hampered by the need to explain what has been going on, to pick up old relationships, to sort out unpaid bills, and so on. Not surprisingly, fear of relapse can have a profound impact on a person's life, inhibiting him/her from taking any risks and causing himself/herself any unnecessary anxiety. However, this also reduces the range of experiences that can be enjoyed, and limits his/her expectations (Strauss 1994). Sometimes a reluctance to undertake any activity that might precipitate frightening symptoms is interpreted as 'lack of motivation' or 'negative symptoms' (Watkins 1996). Such interpretations are pejorative and rarely lead to appropriate solutions.

Surveys of what people want from services repeatedly demonstrate that they want to have control over their symptoms, to be able to predict relapse, and to manage crises (Mueser et al 1992). Many people already recognise the signs of impending relapse and take remedial action (Breier & Strauss 1983, McCandless-Glincher et al 1986, Kumar et al 1989). It is this evidence that individuals can recognise and act on symptoms that has led to the development of 'early interventions' to prevent relapse (Birchwood et al 1998).

Around 60% of people who have experienced a relapse are able to identify the 'early warning signs' that may herald it. Often dysphoria (anxiety, sensitivity, withdrawal) are the first things that a person notices, but everyone has a unique 'personal relapse signature' with different features. With each successive relapse, a person develops a more accurate understanding of his/her own 'signature'. It is important to stress that the 'relapse signature' does not automatically herald a breakdown. Rather, it indicates that the person may be at risk of relapse and is a sign that they may need to do something.

Early intervention: preventing and minimising crises
Assessment
The first step involves the person exploring his/her own 'relapse signature', i.e. the pattern of events, thoughts, feelings and behaviour that may herald problems. It is often helpful to ask the person to think back to the last time he/she experienced problems and go through, step by step, the period over which these developed. Close friends, partners and family members may be able to assist the person in identifying these 'early signs'. Birchwood et al (1998) has developed an 'early signs interview' with five stages: the date of onset of the episode and the time before admission; the date when a change in behaviour was first noticed; the sequence of changes up to relapse; the detailed nature of these changes; and, finally, a summary of the changes.

Monitoring
On the basis of the early warning signs identified, people can then monitor their own experiences. Often people describe problems as coming 'out of the blue'. Such unpredictability can be very distressing and disabling. We have met many people who had ceased to plan anything – going out with friends, booking a holiday, taking a college course – for fear that their problems would suddenly get worse and prevent them from doing what they had planned. If a person can begin to monitor his/her owns 'ups and downs' then it is often possible to detect patterns in them and begin to gain a sense of control. Many people find it helpful to do a kind of 'daily monitoring' of themselves against the early warning signs that they have identified. For example, the Manic Depression Fellowship self-management programmes have developed a diary with a 'traffic-light' system for recording mood swings, where 'amber' indicates early signs of difficulties. Again, some people find it helpful to enlist the assistance of family and close friends to help alert them to emerging difficulties.

Intervention
The information gained during assessment and monitoring can be used to help the person develop a plan of action. Publications are available from

Table 8.1   Relapse warning signs and appropriate actions

Warning signs	Action
Feeling tearful for no reason; becoming irritable with people around me; lack of interest in sex.	Cut down on social engagements. Try to avoid taking on new jobs at work. Stick to a daily routine. Stop drinking alcohol. Make sure I eat properly and go for a walk after work every evening. Explain to my partner that I am not feeling too good.
Waking early in the morning; loss of appetite; great difficulty in keeping going at work.	Make sure that everything is in order at work: write down where I have got to with jobs that I am doing. Ask my partner to take over chores at home. Make an appointment to see the doctor and ask to increase medication.
Unable to go out or drive the car; unable to talk to people; unable to make simple decisions about what to wear; sleeping very little.	Ask partner to: 1. tell work I am sick and tell my friend at work my computer password and where she can find information about where I've got to with the things I'm doing; 2. make an emergency appointment to get me to the hospital and take me there; 3. tell my friends and parents that I am not well.

many mental health organisations, e.g. Mind, Rethink and the Manic Depression Fellowship, which help people to develop plans like this. Many people's 'relapse signature' involves a number of stages, different courses of action being appropriate at each one (Table 8.1).

PLANNING AHEAD

Often a person's plan for preventing and minimising crises requires the co-operation of others (family, friends, colleagues, mental health workers). Some people have found it useful to negotiate ways in which they can trigger more help from services, or to adjust their medication themselves when they begin to experience difficulties. However, when in crisis, many people find such decisions and negotiations difficult, therefore planning ahead is useful so that everyone is aware of the help that is required in the event of problems. Such 'advanced directives' or 'crisis plans' can be very important in reducing the fear associated with crises and should be a central part of each person's care plan. Many people also find it useful to carry a briefer 'crisis card' that indicates who should be contacted in an emergency.

The Manic Depression Fellowship (2001) has produced a useful booklet to help people plan ahead. Although this is intended for people with bipolar disorder, it is equally applicable to those who experience other types of problems. It reminds people to make plans in relation to the following aspects of life.

◆ family, friends and others – explaining what happens, how it feels, what is the 'real me', talking to children about the nature of your problems and planning childcare in advance.

◆ looking after your home – listing practical matters that need looking after (heating, bills, pets), and arranging for friends or neighbours to have a spare set of keys and take over certain matters in a crisis.

◆ employment – deciding what you want your employer and colleagues to know, who will tell them, and how they are to be told.

◆ looking after your money – finding out about benefits and employment rights, and planning for someone to pay regular bills if you become unwell. If you have been inclined to spend too much when becoming ill, it is necessary to work out a way of limiting possible spending, e.g. locking away credit cards and protecting savings by delaying access.

The *Planning Ahead* booklet also provides a useful form for planning care in the event of a hospital admission. This is completed in advance and witnessed/signed by the mental health worker; one copy is kept in the medical notes, another is held by the individual, and it may be useful for a further copy to be held by a close friend. Such plans should give information about behaviour when that person is becoming unwell and the sort of help he/she would like. They should list the treatments that have been helpful in the past (and those that have not) and should include the person's wishes about having these treatments again. They might also include information about special needs, general health, and the people who can be contacted in a crisis – with notes about information that may be given to them. As well as providing guidance in a crisis, this sort of planning can help the mental health worker negotiate what help the person wants from services, and guide the contents of their 'care plan'.

SUPPORTING RELATIONSHIPS WITH FAMILY AND FRIENDS

Relationships are important in and of themselves, but they can also provide the practical and emotional support on which most of us rely in order to do the things we want to do. Serious mental health problems have a profound impact not only on the life of the person who experiences them, but also on his/her family and friends. Mental health workers may have a role to play in supporting a person's family and friends and helping him/her to maintain close relationships. Friends and relations can find it difficult to be with some-one who is extremely distressed and disturbed. Often they feel unsure of what to do for the best, and experience increased strain, worry and distress as well as a diminution in their own social life and contacts (e.g. see Creer et al 1982, Fadden et al 1987, Lefley 1989).

> *What has it been like for us these past 10 years? I will begin with what has always been most painful for me – those feelings of loss, grief and mourn-ing... the loss of the son I once had, because in many ways he is quite dif-ferent..... There is also the terrible loss of our expectations. We feel cheated out of watching him mature and flower the way adolescents do as they grow into young adults..... There is also a loss of some kind of emotional connectedness that is a consequence of some of the negative symptoms.... There is also some inner sense of shame and humiliation that I occasional-ly feel... [although] I have no horror stories to tell about bad treatment and inconsiderate doctors. No one has blamed us for his illness. (Willick 1992)*

The role of families, and the problems they experience, is recognised in Standard 6 of the *Mental Health National Service Framework* (Department of Health 1999). This requires that relatives are involved in the planning of care, and receive help with problems they may have. It is required that their needs are assessed and plans made to provide them with the support and help they need. Despite a recognition that people who are important to the client need emotional support, practical help and information, it remains the case that mental health services have great difficulty in providing these things. Relatives often feel ill-informed and unsupported by staff members who do not recognise the contribution they make and the difficulties they experience. Some feel that members of staff blame them for their relative's problems (Shepherd et al 1995, Winefield & Burnett 1996).

'Expressed Emotion' Approaches

Work with families has developed from an understanding of the 'stress-vulnerability' model described above (see Falloon et al 1982, 1984, Tarrier 1992). Initial reactions to a family member developing serious mental health problems include bewilderment, anxiety, denial and the often over-optimistic expectation that everything will soon 'get back to normal'. When such expec-tations are not realised, and the problems continue, this can lead to frustra-tion, irritation and criticism of the person, or attempts to look after them, compensate for their impairments and take over their social roles ('emotional over-involvement'). These combine to constitute the 'expressed emotion' which is a robust predictor of outcome. People returning to live in high 'expressed emotion' settings are more likely to relapse within the next nine months than those going back to live with families showing low 'expressed emotion'. It is important to remember that high 'expressed emotion' is not restricted to families: criticism and 'emotional over-involvement' are equally prevalent among mental health practitioners, with similar consequences.

A link has also been established between 'expressed emotion' and the 'burden' experienced by family members (Jackson et al 1990, Scazufca & Kuipers 1999): people who find the relationship difficult also find it harder to provide care. The 'expressed emotion' measure may be defined as an assessment of the quality of the relationship, and both 'expressed emotion' and the 'burden' are more dependent on an appraisal of the person's problems than on the social and mental health problems themselves. The situation is made more difficult if the relatives do not have a job or spend excessive amounts of time with the person. Where relatives believe that the person has complete control over their actions, they are likely to deem the person responsible for their difficult behaviours. These may then be attributed to, for example, 'laziness' or 'lack of motivation', and high levels of irritation and criticism are likely to ensue. An understanding of problems which reduces blame can lead to a more positive view of the individual. On the other hand, where relatives see the disabled person as being like a small child – completely incapable and in need of continual supervision – the consequence is likely to be over-involvement.

Kuipers (2001) has built on extensive work with families to list factors that can help them cope. These factors might equally apply to others who are close to the client, and include the following: finding something positive in the person – something that they like about him/her as he/she is now; understanding the difference between 'poor motivation' and 'laziness' so that they blame the person less; taking things slowly and acknowledging small successes; encouraging the person to be as independent as possible; maintaining their own outside interests; and looking after themselves.

In work with families and friends, issues of confidentiality often arise. Clearly, a person's wishes regarding confidentiality must be respected. However, this does not mean that the difficulties experienced by relatives and friends can be ignored: it is possible to address their problems and needs *in their own right* without compromising confidentiality. In order to minimise perceived or actual conflicts of interest, it may be preferable for support of relatives to be provided by someone who is not working directly with the person concerned. On the basis of a 'stress-vulnerability' perspective, a range of family interventions have been developed (Leff & Vaughn 1985, Kuipers & Bebbington 1988, Falloon et al 1984, Tarrier et al 1988). These combine a number of components.

Education about the nature of mental health problems

The most common complaint from families is lack of information. Information can help them to understand the nature of the difficulties that might be expected with serious mental health problems and the different forms of treatment and help available. It is likely that they will have negative or exaggerated images of 'madness' that make it difficult for them to accept its existence in their family. Education can help to dispel these myths and address family members' worst fears and anxieties. It may be useful for them to find out about different theories about mental health problems and their prognoses, as this can assuage their feelings of guilt and blame. Information should be given in a manner that is sensitive to their level of understanding, their 'readiness' to hear, and their interest (they may want to read everything available to find out as much as they can, or they may find it more helpful to receive simple explanations of difficulties as they arise).

Reappraisal of the difficulties the person experiences
As the family members begin to understand the nature of the difficulties experienced by the person, they can be helped to adjust to their problems. Families, like mental health professionals, can both help and hinder a person's recovery. It is important that those close to the person are assisted to understand the person's situation and challenges, rather than blaming him/her. Rather than removing all expectations from the person, they may be helped to negotiate appropriate goals. Rather than seeing the person's life as hopeless and devastated, it is important that they hold out hope, recognize the person's strengths and help him/her to work towards new goals.

Emotional processing of grief and loss
The occurrence of serious mental health problems in a family member or close friend can be very traumatic. People may grieve for the loss of the person they knew, the expectations they had of that person, and the relationship that they once shared. People often find it helpful to talk about these feelings, to share their lost hopes and to hear how other family members feel. The mental health worker may have an important role to play in hearing their stories and acknowledging their anger and despair. However, it is important that workers also offer hope that the person can rebuild a meaningful and valued life and that relationships do not have to be damaged beyond repair. Family and friends, like the person himself/herself, face the challenge of recovery, and understanding their own reactions can be an important component of this journey. Spaniol & Zipple (1994) have identified a number of distinct phases in this family recovery process:

❶ *Discovery/denial.* When family members look for alternative explanations for the behaviour of the person, e.g. drugs, alcohol, laziness, 'adolescence', influence of friends. They may also seek alternative solutions for the problems, e.g. through the church or by changing school. Different members of the family may well accept the possibility of mental health problems at different rates. They each have to understand that everyone in the family will have their own way of coping and will adjust in different ways. There is no wrong or right way of behaving, and emotional reactions may well be intense and distressing.

❶ *Recognition/acceptance.* As the problems persist, the family begins to accept that one of their kin has mental health problems. Initially they may look to professionals for a cure, but if this becomes unlikely then they begin to grieve for lost hopes, expectations and relationships. Often parents' sense of value is contingent upon the 'success' of their offspring – at school, at work, and in relationships. They, too, need to find new sources of possibility and hope.

I'd always expected him to get married and leave home, but as it is we're lucky to still have him around. We've always enjoyed bird watching together and now we can go whenever we like.

I'm so proud of him. He was so ill, and now look – he's out every day working at the centre and he runs errands for me – I can't get up and down the stairs very well you know. (two fathers of sons with diagnoses of schizophrenia, cited in Perkins & Repper 1998)

❶ *Coping.* Grief is overtaken by the reality of the difficulties and the family begins the struggle of managing. They may feel angry, despairing, inadequate and they may reject help from the professionals, whom they see as having failed to provide a solution. Other families with similar experiences, as well as mental health workers, may help in developing coping strategies.

❶ *Personal and political advocacy.* As they recover, families often change: they blame themselves less, they let go of what they can't change, they work out more productive relationships with services, and they may become more assertive and confident about their own role. Some family members may become involved in political action to change the systems of support. Through such action, they may experience, for the first time, their own collective power and influence.

Problem-solving approaches

Families and friends may benefit from the problem-solving framework described earlier in this chapter. The mental health worker may have a role in helping the person and his/her family/friends to negotiate, compromise, work together for their common good, and understand that different family members have different perceptions, priorities and responses.

The effectiveness of these family 'psychosocial' interventions has been demonstrated in numerous studies (Pharoah et al 2001). They have been shown to reduce relapse and readmission rates and to enhance social functioning. However, they have not been without their critics (Perkins & Repper

1998). For example, Hatfield et al (1987) have argued that such theories are not enough of a departure from traditional models that blamed families for mental illness, and that they continue to alienate them from mental health services:

> *Since high EE [expressed emotion] is seen as undesirable, then high EE families may justifiably feel that they have been labeled 'bad families'. Once again the focus is on family deficit and families are viewed negatively ... There is, perhaps, more to be gained from studying the strengths of people rather than their frailties. It is upon strengths that alliances with professionals can be built.*

We are also concerned about the concept of 'burden' that is so prevalent in work with families. For example, Szmuckler (1996) has argued that framing carers' problems in terms of 'burden' is pejorative and unhelpful. As we have already seen, people with mental health problems can, and do, contribute positively to family life (Greenberg et al 1994).

In enabling people with mental health problems to take back control over their lives it is important to remember that no man or woman is an island. Our lives exist in the context of other people – both those who are close to us, such as family and friends, and those who are less close, such as colleagues, neighbours and others with whom we share places and activities. These people all have an important role to play in the recovery journey. We must help people to maintain those roles and relationships that are important to them, as well as assisting them to access new opportunities and social networks. It is towards some of the ways in which this might be achieved that the next section of this book is directed.

Section 3

Facilitating recovery: promoting social inclusion

3

9

Developing services that facilitate access

Although few people with mental health problems now live in large, remote asylums, physically exiled from community life, many remain as excluded as ever. A person's physical presence in a community – whether living in a supported or an independent setting – does not mean that they are included: positively accepted as a part of that community, rather than merely tolerated. Nor does it mean that they are able to access the facilities and opportunities within that community. Too often, the person continues to feel, and be treated as, an outsider. The situation that Esso Leete (1989) describes remains a reality for many:

> *Your college refuses to admit you after discharge because you now have a history of mental illness...you are denied a driver's license because you were stupid enough to answer their questionnaire truthfully...your friends decide they need to develop other friendships upon learning of your past troubles and treatment.*

This list could be extended: the local GP surgery refuses to register you because you may make excessive demands on them; the general hospital does not take your physical health problems seriously; and employers will not consider your application. And, of course, the poverty that ensues from a life on state benefits means that you cannot afford to go out to the pub, travel, go to the cinema, join a sports club, and too often means that you are living in a high crime area where you feel afraid to go out.

Where a person is accepted as part of the local community, there is no guarantee that this will be a positive and valuing acceptance. Sometimes people are allowed to participate because others feel sorry for them, or see them as an object of fun. For example, in a local pub one evening we saw a man with whom we worked. Surprisingly, he was behaving strangely – continually smiling, giggling, wandering from person to person 'playing the fool'. When asked why he was doing this he replied that by 'acting mad' people would speak to him and buy him drinks. When he did not behave in this way he simply sat in the corner, ignored. It seems that the position of 'village idiot' is still available.

Alternatively, people with mental health problems may be given access only to those things that no one else wants. For example, we saw a publicity leaflet which asked employers if they had posts in their business that were 'hard to fill' and that 'no one wants' that they could make available to people with mental health problems on 'transitional employment placements'. ('Transitional employment' is part of the range of opportunities offered by the 'Clubhouse' services for people with mental health problems to help them to get back to open employment.)

Conceptions of 'madness' developed through family lore, personal experience, peer relationships and the media continue to portray people with mental health problems as less trustworthy, less intelligent and less competent than others (Link et al 2001). If the consequences of prejudice and discrimination are assumed to be the consequences of illness, then a self-fulfilling spiral of exclusion ensues. For example, a belief that people with mental health problems are unable to work ensures that 82% of such people are unemployed (National Office of Statistics, UK Labour Force Survey 2000) and this serves to confirm the belief that they are unable to work. Practitioners and employers alike become sceptical about a person's ability to make a success of open employment, which has knock-on effects for that person's confidence and belief in himself/herself. This, in turn, means that such people fail to make use of the skills that they have:

> *I feel less capable, less competent, less worthwhile than a so-called normal person. Inside I feel less competent because people expect me to be less competent…* (Campbell 1989)

Too often, the response of mental health services is to establish separate, segregated opportunities for people with mental health problems. This may arise from a desire to protect people from discrimination, or from a belief that their problems render them incapable of coping in ordinary settings. Whatever the reason, such an approach has resulted in the proliferation of day centres, sheltered workshops, 'drop-in' centres, and social clubs dedicated to the support of people with mental health problems. These places remain segregated despite their physical location in communities.

Such facilities may have their place, but they are rarely socially valued. It is often difficult to find personal meaning and value in something that is devalued by the community in which you live. Does anyone who is not a member of a devalued group ever entertain an ambition to attend a day centre or a sheltered workshop? No – these are reserved for people with mental health problems, learning difficulties, physical impairments and for older people. Is it any wonder that many people do not like to be seen using such facilities? One woman we know attended a day centre within walking distance of her home, but took two buses to get there so that her neighbours did not know she was doing so. It is also the case that the range of opportunities available in segregated settings is very much more restricted than that available outwith the mental health services, and usually skewed to the lower end of the ability range (basic English, basic Maths, simple packing, or assembly work). Sometimes day facilities and sheltered workshops are seen as a route to open employment and engagement in more integrated settings, but, if this is the aim, evidence suggests that they are singularly unsuccessful in achieving it. Segregated settings constitute an end in themselves, rather than a means to an end, for the majority of those who use them (see, for example, Pozner et al 1996).

Research evidence on employment has repeatedly shown that, if provided with the support they need, as many as 60% of people with more serious mental health problems can gain and sustain open employment (Bond et al 1997, 2001, Crowther et al 2001). Similarly, research has shown that, with support, the majority of people with such difficulties can live independently (Meuser et al 1998). In addition, a range of initiatives have shown that people can equally successfully access education (c.f. Unger et al 1991) and a range of social and leisure opportunities.

However, it remains the case that the majority of people with mental health problems do not receive the support they need to access such opportunities. Unless the provision of the support to ensure access becomes an integral and central component of the mental health services it is unlikely that this situation will change. Chapters 11 and 12 discuss the ways in which mental health workers might help people access the roles, activities and facilities they value. The aim of this chapter is to explore ways in which practitioners might create services that promote social inclusion.

AN INCLUSIVE PHILOSOPHY

Developing a 'philosophy of care' in a busy community team or acute ward can seem like an irrelevant diversion – a gesture resulting in nothing more than a sign on the wall that is regarded with cynicism by both staff members and service-users. However, if a mental health service is to promote inclusion, then all the members of the team must be clear about what they are working towards, how they are working, and the values that underpin their work. The development of such a philosophy must involve the whole team so that differences of approach and priority can be acknowledged and negotiated (Peter Bates, unpublished).

Treatment and symptom control represent only one aspect of the help and support that a person needs in order to facilitate their recovery:

> ... *just as diagnosis is only one part of a person's life, so medical treatment is only one part of the support they need – to cope, to recover and to avoid relapse. The other support – by far the largest part – will come from family, friends, schools, employers, faith communities, neighbourhoods – and from opportunities to enjoy the same range of services and facilities within the community as everyone else.* (Department of Health 2001a)

If mental health services are to actively promote the social inclusion that is so essential for recovery, then this must be an explicit and valued part of their work. If treatment and therapy directed towards symptom reduction are given pride of place then other activities are rendered peripheral. In a busy team, peripheral activities tend to be dropped when there is not the time and resources to attend to them. For example, given a choice between giving a person an injection and returning his/her relative's call, the former is likely to receive priority, even though the precise time at which the injection is given is not critical (it could be given later, by members of the night staff), whereas a timely response to relatives may be central to forming a relationship with them and making them feel included.

However, according pride of place to treatment and therapy has another important consequence. If interventions to maintain and develop social engagement are relegated to 'second place' then staff members will not feel valued when they engage in them. Increasingly, staff groups who have traditionally provided practical and social support – people such as nurses, occupational therapists and social workers – are moving towards 'therapy' as their main activity. Many seek to secure recognition and status within services by defining themselves as 'therapists'. If the promotion of access and inclusion is to be recognised as a core activity then they must be valued by everyone at all levels of the service. Unless board members, senior managers and senior clinicians prioritise these activities, direct-care staff members will not see them as central to their work or feel valued for providing them. The success of services must be judged not only in terms of symptomatic improvement and discharge, but also in terms of the number of clients who are able to secure jobs or college courses, the extent to which relatives receive enough information and feel included and supported, the number of people who have a place of their own or engage in social and leisure activities, and the number of relatives and friends who visit the wards. In this context, it is important to note two research findings.

First, promoting access and inclusion is important in improving a person's health as well as their social functioning. Social functioning, psychological well-being, and physical and mental health are intimately interlinked. For example, the absence of social supports and social networks is detrimental to mental health (Simmons 1994). The absence of employment has been linked with increased general health problems, including premature death (Brenner 1979, Smith 1985, Beale & Nethercott 1985, Bartley 1994), and there is a particularly strong relationship between unemployment and mental health difficulties (Smith et al 1993, Warr 1987, Warner 2000). Unemployment is associated with increased use of mental health services (Brenner & Bartell 1983, Wilson & Walker 1993, Warner 1994, Steward 1996) and is known to increase the risk of suicide (Platt & Kreitman 1984, Moser et al 1987, Philippe 1988, Lewis & Sloggett 1998).

Second, the vocational literature shows that, if efforts to promote inclusion are to be successful, then they must be integrated into the clinical work of the team rather than being a separate problem for distinct services (Bond et al 1997, 2001). For example, decisions about the prescribing of medication and about helping people to return to work must be interlinked: side-effects may impair a person's ability to work, and the week before a person returns to work is not the time to make changes in medication.

If the promotion of social inclusion is to be valued, then it must be a central part of the aims, ambitions and values of the organisation as a whole, as well as the 'philosophy of care' of individual units. In order to promote recovery, the philosophy of a service – whether it be a community team, in-patient ward, day hospital or resource centre – should be inclusive in a number of ways:

◆ inclusive of a social perspective – the person's roles and relationships as well as their symptoms
◆ inclusive of a person's strengths and abilities, and identifying, maintaining and promoting these
◆ inclusive of those people who are important in the person's life (e.g. family, friends, employers, teachers) and supporting these relationships
◆ inclusive of the way in which a person copes with the experience of his/her mental health problems and enabling him/her to take control of these difficulties
◆ inclusive of the person's own aspirations and goals, and helping him/her to pursue them.

INCLUSIVE PRACTICES

Standard 1 of the *Mental Health National Service Framework* (Department of Health 1999) specifically requires that services reduce the discrimination experienced by people with mental health problems. This may be achieved in a number of ways. An increasing number of 'anti-stigma' and 'anti-discrimination' initiatives have been established by organisations such as the World

Health Organisation, the World Psychiatric Association, the Royal College of Psychiatrists and the Department of Health, as well as voluntary organisations such as Mind. However, a great deal can be done to promote inclusion by mental health workers at the level of the individual team.

Promoting inclusion is not the province of a particular profession, which does not mean that traditional professional skills are unimportant, but it does mean that these skills need to be used in the service of helping the client to maintain or regain valued roles and relationships. If, for example, a person wishes to return to work, pharmacological, psychological, occupational and social interventions can be tailored towards this end:

◆ In considering the optimal type, dosage and timing of medication, symptom control must be balanced against specific side-effects that may make work difficult. A person may be able to work if he/she continues to experience some auditory hallucinations, but will be unable to do so if he/she is extremely drowsy in the morning.

◆ Psychological interventions can be directed towards helping the person to identify specific problems and symptoms that might cause difficulties at work, and to developing strategies for dealing with these things in a particular work situation. In Chapter 8, we have seen some of the ways in which Esso Leete (1989) has achieved this. For example, 'If I do become overwhelmed in a social situation, I may temporarily withdraw by going into another room (even the restroom) to be alone for a while.'

◆ Occupational interventions might be directed towards helping a person to maintain and enhance the specific skills he/she needs for work. For example, a secretary might benefit from the opportunity to practice typing or computing skills while in an in-patient facility.

◆ Social interventions might be directed towards helping a person to maintain contact with his/her employer. This would include basic necessities like making sure that they have sent in a 'sickness certificate', helping the person to speak with his/her manager to find out how he/she is doing, and when he/she might be able to return. Help might involve, for example, negotiating a graded return to work, having an opportunity to get 'up to speed' on what has happened while he/she was away (by meeting the manager before returning or taking papers home), working out what to tell colleagues about why he/she has been away, and helping him/her actually to get in to work on the first day back.

This type of multidisciplinary approach specifically tailored to maximising someone's chances of maintaining or gaining access to valued roles and activities applies in both in-patient and out-patient settings and to all the areas of that person's life and social network. For example, if a person has been in hospital, it is important to help him/her resume those things that he/she values. This may include taking up family roles and parental responsibilities, getting back to helping in the local church, making contact with friends, and going back to college or the local football team.

Promoting inclusion is not simply about enabling people to engage in the activities they want. Critically, it also involves maintaining and promoting important relationships with friends, family and others who are important in the person's life. Sustaining and developing such relationships involves helping both the individual and these other people. Friends can feel unsure about how to help. They, too, need to understand what has happened and how to respond to behaviour that may seem to them confusing and uncharacteristic. They may feel unwelcome when they visit the person in hospital, or frightened by his/her behaviour. They may withdraw from the person because they feel uncertain about what to do and are fearful of making matters worse. They may feel rejected if the person fails to contact them or pushes them away. A person may do this because he/she is too distressed, is uncomfortable about telling other people what has happened, or is embarrassed about friends and relations seeing him/her when he/she is having difficulties. In a Mental Health Foundation (2001) survey of 421 friends of people who had experienced mental health problems, 58% said that they needed support themselves if they were to support their friend.

Employers, colleagues, teachers, people from the local church, or others with whom the person has contact, may well be in a similar position. The person may have behaved in ways which they find confusing, frightening or irritating. Alternatively, the person may have simply 'disappeared' when he/she developed problems, for example failed to turn up for work, college or church, and was thus seen as 'letting down' others. However much they may want to help, unless they have an understanding of what is going on, the person's contacts may find it difficult to know what to do to include the person and welcome him/her back. Support for those who share places and activities with the person can greatly enhance his/her opportunities for participation.

It is hard to tell other people that you have 'gone mad'. Often, people need help to explain what has happened. They may appreciate it if the mental health worker makes initial contact for them and explains what has happened. One woman with whom we worked asked us to meet with her son and herself to explain why she had been 'different' lately, because she did not feel able to tell him on her own. Some people might prefer to tell others themselves – by writing a letter, telephoning, or arranging to meet – but they may value help in working out what to say and how much detail to give. If others visit the person in hospital, they may well be apprehensive. The mental health worker can make things easier by welcoming them and perhaps helping them to understand why the person may be behaving as he/she does (Hutchinson & Nettle 2001). Sometimes it may be necessary to arrange transport for visitors if they are to maintain contact.

In giving information to a person's friends, family and social contacts, issues of confidentiality are an important consideration. While the person may not want staff to talk to other people about his/her problems, treatment and support, it is possible to do a number of things:

◆ It is possible to discuss, with the person, what he/she does and does not want others to know – the provision of information is not an 'all or nothing' thing.

◆ The mental health worker could discuss, how the person would like people to be given the information he/she wishes them to have. Perhaps he/she would prefer to tell them himself/herself (with or without the help of the mental health worker), or write a letter, or check the contents of a letter written by the practitioner. There are numerous possibilities.

◆ More general information about different psychiatric problems, their treatment, and the services available could be provided.

◆ The mental health worker could talk, in general terms, about why different types of difficulty might arise, and how they might be addressed ('Many people with mental health problems feel . . . .', 'There are a number of ways of dealing with the sort of problems you describe . . .').

◆ The practitioner could address the problems that friends and family and other social contacts are having – including the person's reluctance to share information with them and the possible reasons for this – and provide them with help and support in their own right.

The chorus of complaints about the dearth of information continues from both people with mental health problems and their friends and relatives (Shepherd et al 1995, Read & Reynolds 1996, Campbell & Lindow 1997, Faulkner & Layzell 2000, Rose 2001, Mental Health Foundation 2001). Rose (2001) has shown that the quality of information provided is a major determinant of people's overall satisfaction with services. However, information is equally critical for others who are important in the person's life if they are to accept, accommodate, and support him/her. Information can be provided in a number of ways:

◆ Information may be produced by mental health workers, voluntary or community groups and service-user's or relatives' organisations.

◆ It may be available within mental health services (hospitals, clinics, day centres/hospitals, carers' centres), in places within the local community (GP surgeries, local libraries, community centres, advice centres, local shops and supermarkets, etc.) and/or in various publications that are widely read (local papers, the magazines that employers and teachers/lecturers regularly read, etc.).

◆ It may be provided in written form, verbally or electronically. A great deal of useful information can be conveyed in one-to-one interactions with the mental health worker, but it can also be conveyed via seminars and talks to, for example, local employers and employment organisations, local schools, community groups, faith communities, relatives' meetings and user/survivor groups. Increasingly, people are finding out about health problems for themselves by using the internet. Practitioners have a role in directing them towards helpful sites.

Any information provided should fulfil certain criteria:

◆ The information must be jargon free, clear and straightforward. Not only should it avoid complex technical terminology, it should also avoid those terms that, while used routinely in the mental health services, mean little to those outside – terms such as 'care-programme approach' and 'care co-ordinator'.

◆ The material should be available in a variety of languages and formats (e.g. tape, Braille and easy-read).

◆ The information should be easily accessible in both format and style. It should be presented in a 'user-friendly' form and should not be too long: few people will wade through pages and pages of closely typed script.

◆ The material should be provided in easily accessible places, both within and outwith mental health services.

◆ The information must be appropriate to the people for whom it is designed, i.e. relevant and tailored to the needs of different audiences. For example, details of diagnosis, symptomatology, aetiology, prognosis and treatment are not usually of great concern to employers. They want to know whether the person will turn up for work and be reliable, whether he/she can do the job, specific problems that the person may have at work, the sort of adjustments others in the workplace might have to make, and what sort of help is available for both employer and employee should they need it. Relatives, on the other hand, are typically interested in knowing about different disorders/problems, prognosis, treatments and interventions, and the different supports and services available (including where they can get help in an emergency). A number of organisations have produced information specifically tailored for different audiences, e.g. the Employers' Forum of Disability (www.employers-forum.co.uk), Mind (www.mind.org.uk), the Manic Depression Fellowship (www.mdf.org.uk), The Mental Health Foundation (www.mental-health.org.uk/), the Royal College of Psychiatrists (www.rcpsych.ac.uk/)/and Rethink (www.rethink.org.uk).

Finally, and most importantly, inclusive practices must involve service-users at all levels, from individual care planning and delivery (through the operation and evaluation of individual teams and facilities) to the planning and development of mental health services. These issues are addressed in Chapter 12.

AN INCLUSIVE ENVIRONMENT

While an inclusive philosophy, approach and practices are all important, the extent to which a service is able to facilitate access and promote inclusion is also influenced by the physical environment in which it operates. The environment is particularly important in acute and day facilities, but it can also influence the way in which out-patient facilities and other community services function. Many of the structural aspects of in-patient and community facilities are hardly conducive to maintaining contact. Places that are remote, segregated, difficult to find, poorly signposted and without an obvious reception desk are all unwelcoming. Peeling paint and an environment devoid of pictures and plants convey to people using the service that they are not valued, respected or seen as important. They also make the place unpleasant and unwelcoming for visitors.

Many people have never been inside a psychiatric facility, and maintain 'One Flew Over the Cuckoo's Nest' images of straightjackets and the like. These images are reinforced if you are not sure about the visiting times or arrangements, if you have to wait ages before someone answers the door bell and demands who you are and what you want, and if you have to meet your friend or relative in a smoke-filled, crowded day room with the television blaring. It is unsurprising that many friends and relatives are reluctant to visit. As one friend said, '[I felt] shocked and worried. Appalled at the state of the hospital. Felt as if my friend had died and I was grieving for them.' (cited in Mental Health Foundation Report 2001) Enabling people to maintain contact with each other during an in-patient admission is particularly important, but it is also something which practitioners in out-patient and community settings must take seriously. While it may be difficult for practitioners to make substantial changes to the structure of the physical environment in which services operate, there are a number of things that they can do to make them more acceptable and accessible. These could include:

◆ Putting up a few direction signs (even if these are simply printed out on cards, as may happen for a conference or meeting) so that the place is easy to find.

◆ Making sure that someone is responsible for answering telephones and making visitors welcome. Perhaps a member of staff on each shift could be allocated this task, or, if no receptionist is available, team members could take it in turn on a rota basis.

◆ Finding out about the people who are important in the person's life and to actively encourage them to make contact. This may be done by, for example, inviting them to visit the ward and meet the doctor/care co-ordinator or by sending them information about visiting times and help that may be available to them.

◆ Making sure that the operation and procedures of services are explained to relatives, friends and visitors, and that they know the identity of key personnel such as the ward or team manager, the consultant, and the person's care co-ordinator or key nurse. Up-to-date notice-boards can be useful in this regard.

◆ Prominently displaying useful information leaflets in wards, clinics and resource centres. These might provide information about mental health difficulties and the help available, as well as details of non-mental health facilities, supports and events in the local area.

◆ Facilitating visiting by offering to arrange transport, helping with child-care, and offering appointments to meet key personnel at times that are convenient to people who may be working.

◆ Helping people in hospital to go and visit their friends and relatives outside.

◆ Providing training to ensure that practitioners are aware of the needs of relatives, friends, employers, etc., and to increase confidence in communicating with them.

◆ Making small changes to improve the environment, such as putting up pictures or posters, or acquiring a few plants, books, newspapers and magazines.

◆ Ensuring that enough ash trays are always available to reduce the likelihood of cigarette burns on carpets.

◆ Providing people with access to kitchens where they can make refreshments for themselves and their visitors; 'staff-only' toilets and sitting-rooms should be abolished.

◆ Finding a room in which people can meet visitors in private. Perhaps one of the consulting rooms or meeting rooms could serve this function when it is not being used for other purposes.

◆ Providing refreshments for visitors and for people waiting for appointments.

◆ Making it possible for clients to do things with their visitors, e.g. by providing board-games, cards, toys for children, and magazines for people to read.

◆ Spending time talking to visitors, or relatives and friends who come to out-patient appointments, to address any concerns that they may have.

◆ Moving the telephone to a place where people can talk in private.

◆ Providing writing materials, envelopes and stamps so that people can write to relatives, friends and others with whom they wish to maintain contact.

◆ Reporting faults, damage and breakages promptly; staff members should make a point of 'chasing' maintenance departments to ensure that repairs are done as soon as possible.

◆ Making regular checks to ensure that the place is clean, that there is toilet paper in the toilets, and that there are the materials necessary for making drinks and snacks in the kitchen.

◆ Advising (along with service-users and their relatives) on the design of new units and facilities to ensure that they are accessible (for example, that they have proper reception areas, waiting rooms and visiting rooms, that they are located in a place that is easy to get to, and that they have floor-coverings that are resistant to spillages and cigarette burns).

Facilitating access and promoting inclusion always involve according priority to three areas: helping the individual to access those roles, relationships and activities that he/she values; supporting, and making it possible for, people who are important in a person's life to maintain contact; and increasing the capacity of community facilities and opportunities to accommodate and meet the needs of people who experience mental health problems. In this chapter, we have considered the ways in which services might be organised in order to promote inclusion. In the next two chapters we look at some of the ways in which practitioners can facilitate inclusion.

10

Facilitating access for the individual

INTRODUCTION

Almost everywhere they turn, people with mental health problems encounter barriers that stand in the way of their being able to do what they want to do. Cognitive and emotional problems make it more difficult to do things that others take for granted. It can, for example, be difficult to concentrate on what other people are saying if you also have to contend with a chorus of private and competing voices within your head commenting on your every word and action. However, people with such difficulties can, and do, work out ways of living with these things. More difficult are the ways in which such experiences are viewed by other people, the discrimination that people encounter in all areas of their lives, and the devastating impact of such prejudice on their own self-confidence.

Counteracting exclusion by facilitating access to valued opportunities is essential to recovery and must therefore be a central part of our work. There are a number of general issues that every mental health worker must consider: How can we maintain what they already have? How can we develop new possibilities? How can we make links with local communities? How can we help these local communities become more receptive and inclusive of people with mental health problems? Should people tell others about their problems? These issues are discussed in this chapter.

MAINTAINING WHAT A PERSON ALREADY HAS

In mental health services we are often so concerned about people's symptoms that we fail to notice other things that are important in their lives. Only later, when many contacts have been lost, do we turn our attention to 'rehabilitation' and helping them to resume activities. The cost of this in terms of lost opportunities and the erosion of hope is incalculable.

If we are to promote inclusion, efforts to maintain a person's connections through a period of mental health difficulties are an important facet of the work of both primary and secondary mental health services. For most people who develop mental health problems, their first contact is with the GP; some people will receive all the treatment they need at a primary care level. Problems such as anxiety and depression have led to the loss of many jobs and relationships, so the role of primary care in promoting social inclusion should not be underestimated. We would not wish to see resources directed away from those with more enduring and disabling difficulties. However, attention to the maintenance of social and vocational connections should be a standard part of the treatment of 'mild to moderate' mental health problems in primary care. Initiatives such as Prescriptions for Learning, developed by the National Institute for Adult Continuing Education, and the introduction of vocational advisors into GP surgeries are positive developments in this regard.

Within secondary services, the developing Early Intervention Teams (Department of Health 2001c) are going some way to addressing the maintenance of social roles, relationships and activities at an early stage. This work cannot be seen as the province of any one specialist service; it must be a central facet of the mental health system as a whole and must begin with a person's first contact with services. Initial assessments should include consideration of the things that the person considers to be important in life, including family and intimate relationships, friendships, employment or education, voluntary work, leisure and sporting activities, social activities, religious and spiritual activities. Attention must then be paid to enabling the person to maintain contact with these things/people through his/her period of mental health difficulties. Even when a person has had mental health problems for some time, it is essential that mental health workers take time to find out about, and help the person to maintain, existing relationships and activities as well as helping him/her to develop new ones.

This is likely to involve a combination of letting people know what has happened, enabling a person to maintain contact even though they may not be able to engage fully, and helping him/her to resume social contacts and activities as soon as he/she can. The person does not have to be fully 'better' in order to resume activities. He/she may well be able to start some things in a graduated and supported way at a very early stage. For example, a person may be able to go out and visit friends, go to church, or start doing bits and pieces of work while he/she is still an in-patient.

Existing relationships and activities constitute an important foundation for the building of new ones. Support from family and friends can, for example, be critical in helping a person to explore other vocational, social and leisure activities. Many people find new friends and hear about work and other opportunities from people they already know and contacts they already have. Although the maintenance of existing connections is important, this does not mean that people do not also want to explore new possibilities.

DEVELOPING NEW POSSIBILITIES . . . BUT WHAT?

Before we can help someone to access opportunities, it is essential to find out what he/she wants to do. We know from the vocational literature that people are more likely to gain and sustain jobs and courses that they *want* to do rather than those that the practitioner thinks they ought to do (see Becker & Drake 1993, Bond et al 1997, 2001). It seems likely that a similar principle applies to other social activities, leisure pursuits and relationships. A person is unlikely to accept help, or persist in his/her efforts, to do something that he/she does not want to do. Indeed, the very essence of recovery is to enable the person to rebuild a life that is *valuable and meaningful to him/her.*

Sometimes people have a clear idea about what it is they want to do, but most of us find it difficult to think beyond the things with which we are immediately familiar; the idea of change is daunting to most of us. When people's connections and activities have been depleted and their confidence sapped, making decisions about what they want to do can be doubly difficult. Choices are inevitably limited by our visions of what is possible; we can only choose that which we know something about. Therefore the first step is often to help people to see what is available in the different arenas of life. Listings magazines offer numerous possibilities. Faith communities often have a range of opportunities on offer. Local newspapers and libraries give all sorts of information about jobs, leisure and social opportunities. For some people, publications directed towards specific ethnic groups, women or the lesbian and gay community may contain information about things that are of interest. The prospectus of any local college gives information about a huge range of educational possibilities that the person may not have thought about. Volunteer bureaux and job centres offer another range of possibilities, and local councils often have directories of a wide variety of groups and organisations that exist. The internet, of course, offers a seemingly limitless range of options.

It is important that we not only enable people to gain access to these sources of information, but also help people to navigate their way around them to find things that may be in line with their interests and ambitions. However, a few lines in a listings magazine or a job advertisement rarely give us all the information we need to decide whether we want to do something. There are a number of ways in which people can find out more details about opportunities they may wish to pursue:

◆ Phoning or writing for more detailed written information (job descriptions, course prospectuses, leaflets about what is on offer at the local leisure centre, and so forth)

◆ Talking to someone, e.g. the Disability Employment Advisor at the local job centre, or a tutor at the local college, who has specialist knowledge of the area

   ◆ Meeting others who have engaged in those activities

   ◆ Visiting different facilities to see what they are like

◆ Experimenting: there are various ways of trying things out, e.g. by work experience, through 'taster sessions' at local sports centres and colleges, or by simply going along with someone to see what it is like.

Finally, it is important to remember that the impact of mental health problems, and all the negativity and discrimination that surround them, may mean that people lack confidence in their ability to manage any new activity; they may look to mental health workers for reassurance. When a person says 'I don't think I can do that.', he/she may be making an informed choice, but he/she may also be reflecting a lack of self-belief. While not wishing to push someone beyond their limits, or into something they do not want to do, it may sometimes be sensible for the practitioner to challenge (gently) the person's decision in order to demonstrate confidence in him/her. If others have confidence in you, then you can begin to develop confidence in yourself. For example, the mental health worker may reply, 'Are you sure? I think you might be able to do that, you know. You are good at ... and you have always enjoyed ...' and perhaps offer to help the person to make a visit, or have a go, or meet someone who is already involved. Such challenges have been important in most people's lives. How many of us would have failed to apply for a new job, start a course, or ask someone to go out with us if we had not had friends and allies around who had given us a firm (but gentle) push?

Providing information and encouragement are not the only ways of helping a person think about what they want to do. Other things may also be useful:

◆ Chart their current activities and help them to think about what aspects of these they enjoy, find valuable, or at which they are successful and those they dislike or are less successful with. This may provide clues to other things they might enjoy.

◆ Examine any difficulties they may have in their current activities; sometimes these can be alleviated by the provision of additional help.

◆ Explore things that they have done in the past and which they may have found rewarding (by looking at their work history, educational achievements, sporting or religious activities and affiliations, etc.). Some of these may be things that they would like to take up again.

◆ Examine the help they have previously received in pursuing these activities: sometimes a lack of success may have resulted from a lack of sufficient support or encouragement.

◆ Consider what family and friends think about the person's ambitions. If those around you do not support what you want to do then this adds to your problems. It may be necessary to work with a person's social network in order to facilitate their engagement.

◆ Explore specific problems and vulnerabilities that might make some types of activity difficult, as this may help to exclude some possibilities.

◆ Delineate the person's existing skills and the things that these might equip him/her to do.

BUT IT'S UNREALISTIC . . .

When a mental health worker looks at a person's problems and life circumstances it is easy to think that his/her wishes and ambitions are unachievable. How many of us can honestly say that our own ambitions have always seemed realistic to others? How many of us, as teenagers, really entertained the ambition of being where we are now? At age 13, R.P. wanted to be the Prime Minister or the captain of a ship, and J.R. wanted to be a showjumper. As we set off in search of our dreams, we did things, things happened, we met people, and different opportunities presented themselves. As a result, our aspirations became modified and we changed direction. We may not have done the things of which we dreamed as teenagers, but in pursuit of them we have achieved a great deal that has been of value. Had our dreams been shattered by the disbelief of others, I wonder whether either of us would be where we are today? How many of us still entertain secret ambitions for the future that no one without 'money to burn' would bet on us achieving (to climb Anna Purna maybe, or to be a member of the House of Lords, or help homeless people in Mexico)? Our dreams and ambitions may have been, and continue to be, unrealistic, but that does not decrease their importance as motivating forces that have given, and continue to give, our lives meaning.

As mental health workers, however, how many dreams and ambitions have we challenged and how much hope have we eroded in our efforts to encourage people to 'be realistic' about their problems and possibilities? The important thing about ambitions and dreams is not their plausibility, but their ability to give direction and meaning to our endeavours. So when someone says he/she wants to be a brain surgeon, or run a record company, perhaps we would be better advised to help him/her to think about how he/she can get there, rather than making judgments about whether he/she ever will get there. For example, we worked with a man who, at the age of 50, had been in hospital continuously for 25 years. He had largely given up hope, and spent most of his days doing very little – rejecting all exhortations to go to 'occupational therapy'. He told us of the time when he had worked as an entertainer at a holiday camp and had dreamed of being a famous musician, and how he loved listening to singers on the radio and imagining that he was one of them. There can be few long-stay psychiatric patients who have become lauded musicians, so his dreams could have been seen as unrealistic, but when we helped him to acquire a mouth-organ he started playing it enthusiastically. He soon bought himself a guitar and started singing. To our untrained ears he lacked a certain 'star quality'. Looking in the local paper, he found information about a folk club in a nearby pub, and we helped him to get there. For months he did not dare to play there, but eventually he did have a go. No, he is not a famous musician, but he does regularly sing in folk clubs and in the local church. He has left hospital, and, although he returns from time to time, his life at the age of 55 is quite different from what it was five years previously. Like so many aspiring musicians, he still dreams that one day he will be 'discovered'. Meanwhile, his life has developed meaning and purpose, he has friends, and does things that he enjoys.

In order to enable people to do the things they want to do, it is important that the mental health services forge greater links with opportunities in the local community.

INFORMATION ABOUT WHAT IS OUT THERE

It is not possible to help people to access opportunities outside the mental health system unless we know what is available. Every mental health service needs to make sure that it has comprehensive information about local opportunities. This must include not only details of facilities specialising in helping people with mental health problems, but also information about things that are available to non-disabled citizens. This might include local colleges, employment opportunities, local sports and leisure facilities, libraries, cinemas, clubs, local places of worship and religious observance, social opportunities, self-help groups, listings magazines, local papers, programmes for local arts and leisure centres, and advice services such as law centres, citizens' Advice Bureaux and disability employment advisors at the job centre.

Staff members who live in the local area often have a wealth of expertise about what is available. Indeed, one of the skills that should be available in the 'skill mix' of any team should be 'local intelligence'. However, if information is to be effective in facilitating access, it must move beyond lists of available opportunities to provide details about what the opportunities and activities are like and what they involve. It is difficult to decide that you want to work in a shop, or study at college, or go to a library without having an idea of what these involve.

Even staff members who live in the local area are unlikely actually to have visited all that is available there. Therefore it is vital that practitioners go and see for themselves by actually visiting local organisations and facilities and finding out who uses them and how they operate so that they are able to tell others about them. For example, a practitioner may go down to the local library and find out how to join it, get a library card, and borrow books. They can collect information such as what identification you need in order to join the library, what information you have to fill in on the form to join, whether you get your library card straight away or have to go back and collect it later, what happens if you lose your card, how long you can borrow books for, what the fines are if books are returned late, and how you can renew a book.

BRIDGE-BUILDING: MAKING LINKS IN THE LOCAL COMMUNITY

In order to enable people to access local opportunities, we, as practitioners, need to create links with different facilities and organisations. Since it is often difficult for one person to have in-depth information about all the opportunities available, it can be helpful for a specific team member to make links actively with a particular sector. The Community Connections Project in Nottingham employed 'bridge-builders' who developed expertise and relationships in the specific domains of spiritual and leisure activities, volunteering and employment, and education. Each of these workers provided individually tailored support to enable people to access opportunities in the areas in which they specialised.

Effective 'bridge-building' involves more than just knowledge of what is available. It means keeping in regular contact with key people, and understanding what these places are like to use, the demands that they make on those who use them, and the sort of people who use them. For example, one 40-year-old woman with whom we worked wanted to go swimming, but was conscious of being somewhat overweight and embarrassed about being seen in her swimsuit. A staff member who had links with local leisure centres was able to tell her about a 'women-only' session on a Saturday afternoon, and an 'aquarobics' class which was frequented by a number of people who were also overweight. She also was able to advise that evenings after school were probably best avoided as the pool tended to be rather crowded with young people.

Making personal links with people involved in local organisations can be very important in increasing their willingness to accommodate those with mental health problems.

BUILDING THE INCLUSIVE CAPACITY OF LOCAL COMMUNITIES

Given the popular myths and misapprehensions that abound, many community facilities are wary about including people who have mental health problems. Even where people are relatively sympathetic, they often feel anxious about how they will cope ('I'm not a mental health expert: I won't know what to do.', 'We're lecturers, not psychiatrists.' and so on).

It is very easy for mental health practitioners to feel overwhelmed by the negative attitudes they encounter within the community and to conclude that until public attitudes have changed there is no hope of service-users ever being accepted. Although prejudice and discrimination are very real barriers, there are many things that mental health workers can do to promote access. Research suggests that a variety of different approaches are generally necessary in order to increase the capacity of community facilities to accommodate people with mental health problems (Warner 2000). In our experience the following principles may be effective:

◆ Promote the inclusion of individuals not illnesses. It is usually more effective to facilitate access for a specific individual rather than for a 'class' of people. If we ask an employer or college to take on 'schizophrenics' we are unlikely to be successful. If we introduce a particular person, emphasise the qualities that fit him/her for the job or course over and above any problems they might have, then people are more likely to accept him/her. People who have experienced mental health problems are their own best advocates. Actually meeting (working with, studying alongside) someone with such difficulties is likely to be more powerful in shaping attitudes than being told about 'them' (c.f. Repper et al 1997).

◆ Explain the problems that a person might experience in ordinary everyday terms as they apply in the particular situation rather than giving details of diagnosis, symptomatology, treatment and prognosis. In describing a person's difficulties, it is helpful to describe their needs and the ways in which these might be met in relation to the specific situation or activity. For example, the person may not be able to stay in church for the whole service, so if he/she sits on the end of a row then it will not disturb other people if he/she has to go out. If someone has difficulty if there are a lot of people around, it would be helpful if another person in the class could go to the canteen with him/her at lunch-time. Perhaps a person tends to get panicky if he/she does not know what to do; writing the instructions down, or explaining who to ask if he/she is unsure is usually helpful. It can be helpful to demystify mental health problems by drawing parallels with the needs of other people. For example, people with mental health problems may benefit from flexibility in working hours – as do employees with care responsibilities. They may need time off for doctors' appointments just like someone who is doing a college course. They may lack confidence just like anyone who has been out of work for some time. We have also found it useful to emphasise that people are not 'ill' all the time, i.e. that their problems may remit completely or fluctuate, and that most of the time most people are able to cope well.

◆ Provide people with opportunities to talk openly about their concerns and past experiences of people with mental health problems so that these can be addressed. Provide practical advice about what to do if they start 'behaving oddly', are 'always off sick', 'disrupt the class', and so forth.

◆ Provide a contact point for use in the event of problems. Many employers, college staff and those running community facilities feel more confident in accommodating people with mental health problems if they know who they can call if they need advice or support. Ideally this should be someone they already know (perhaps a care co-ordinator or link-worker).

◆ It is generally preferable to target particular areas rather than trying to change the whole world: work with lecturers at one college; meet employers at the local chamber of commerce; or provide awareness training and support for young people at the local school. On the basis that direct personal contact is most powerful in changing attitudes, such work should involve people who themselves have experienced mental health problems (especially those who have already been successful in that respect, e.g. someone with mental health problems who is now working, studying, etc.).

In decreasing the myths that surround mental health problems, the provision of information can be critical. There are a number of publications available directed towards people and organisations outside the mental health arena (see, for example, www.mind.org, www.mdf.org.uk, www.niace.org.uk, www.rethink.org, www.rcpsych.ac.uk, and www.employers-forum.co.uk). Employers and service-providers, as well as people with mental health problems, can also obtain information and advice from the Disability Rights Commission (www.drc-gb.org).

ON THE QUESTION OF DISCLOSURE

Engaging in almost any activity outside the mental health services presents people with dilemmas about disclosure of their mental health problems: whether to tell or not to tell, and, if telling, when, how, and whom to tell? Mental health workers often assume that it is 'best' for people to 'be honest' about their problems and so advise them to do so. Ironically, when they have mental health problems themselves, many fail to take this advice. There are numerous mental health professionals who keep very quiet about their mental health problems at work. 'Coming out' is a personal decision. It is, after all, that person, not the practitioner, who has to live with the consequences of the decision he/she makes.

The role of the practitioner should only be to help the person to think through whether he/she wishes to disclose mental health difficulties or not, and help weigh up the advantages and disadvantages of so doing (see Hutchinson & Nettle 2001). Some of the possible pros and cons of disclosure that people might want to think about can be seen in Table 10.1. Although these relate specifically to employment, similar considerations might apply in a range of other situations.

If a person does decide to be open about his/her difficulties in a particular situation, there are many different ways of doing this. People may find it helpful to think through some of these with the mental health worker before deciding what to do. For example, some people prefer to tell only those whom they trust – but once they have told one person, it is difficult to stop others from finding out. Alternatively, they can tell everyone all at once – make a 'grand announcement'. This means that everyone is aware of the difficulties and it decreases the likelihood of inaccurate gossip and rumours. On the other hand, people often find it difficult to know how to respond to 'grand announcements', and there may be some people that they do not wish to trust with this information. Equally, this approach may mean that people see the difficulties as the most important thing about them and lose sight of their other abilities and characteristics. Some clients prefer to get to know people first before they tell them, but it can be difficult to decide when the time is right. Some people prefer to drop it casually into the conversation rather than making a 'big thing' of it. If the person can talk about the problems as if they were the most ordinary thing in the world, then it can be easier for others to accept them as 'no big deal'. It can be very difficult, however, to be casual about doing something that feels like a 'big thing'. The person might want to tell people about all the details of his/her problems, or he/she might prefer to keep these private and talk in more general terms.

Once again, there is no single, optimal way of 'coming out', and it is not the place of mental health workers to prescribe what the person should do. Instead, they can help people to think through the different options, review how they have handled things like this in the past, and learn from their own previous experience. It may also be important to 'normalise' the dilemmas that a person may have and to emphasise that others experience similar difficulties, and that they are not restricted to people with mental health problems. For example, people with HIV/AIDs and lesbians or gay men face similar dilemmas.

Mental health workers are not the only people who can be helpful in making such decisions. As in other areas, people may find the advice of those who

Table 10.1. Some of the pros and cons of disclosure of mental health problems at work

Disadvantages	Advantages
You may be less likely to get the job. (A survey conducted by the Department of Work and Pensions in 2001 showed that, if they faced labour shortages, only 37% of employers would even consider employing someone who had experienced mental health problems.)	If you don't tell your employer you have mental health problems and they find out later they may sack you for lying. If you have not told them about your problems you may not be protected from this kind of discrimination under the Disability Discrimination Act (1995).
If you have already got a job, you may be sacked, or fail to get promotion, if you say you've got mental health problems.	The Disability Discrimination Act (1995) says that employers have to make any 'reasonable adjustments' necessary for you to do the job (e.g. adjustments in hours or parts of the job or working conditions). You cannot ask for such adjustments if you have not been open about your mental health problems.
Your employer may not trust you with responsible jobs.	
If you ask for help with something at work, colleagues may think that you cannot cope because of your mental health difficulties.	You may not have to hide any difficulties you have and may be able to ask for help, time off or a reduced work load at times when you are having difficulties.
You may have to be twice as good as anyone else to prove that you can do the job.	You can ask the employer for time off to go to things such as appointments with doctors.
Every time you have a bad day, or get cross or upset, colleagues may think – that this is because of your mental health problems and conclude that you are not up to the job (even if the problems you are experiencing are perfectly ordinary difficulties that might affect the work of anyone)	You can be honest with your colleagues – it can be very difficult hiding things all of the time.
	If you don't tell your colleagues and they find out, they may gossip behind your back.
Your colleagues may treat you differently if they know you have mental health problems – they may be awkward with you, gossip about you behind your back, not want to be friends with you, or not trust you.	If you tell people about your problems then you will be helping other people with similar difficulties. If your employer can see you are able to do the job, they may be more likely to employ someone else with mental health problems. You can help break down some of the prejudiced attitudes of your colleagues, and enable others who have similar difficulties to talk about them.

have faced similar decisions to be helpful. Others find it useful to talk things through with people with whom they are close, such as friends, partners and family. Yet the experience of mental health problems can leave people very socially isolated, lacking friends and partners with whom they can share their experiences and opinions. This is another aspect of social inclusion in which mental health workers can provide support.

MAKING FRIENDS

Ideally, mental health workers should aim to help people to maintain or resume existing friendships, but there are times when these have already been lost, or cannot be sustained. Repeated surveys testify to the loneliness and isolation of many people with mental health problems, and to the importance that they attach to finding friendships and intimate relationships. It is not uncommon for mental health practitioners to feel unable to meet peoples' needs for friends and partners. Some see it as beyond their professional remit ('I'm not a dating agency'), but friendships and relationships are central to recovery and therefore do constitute part of our work. There are a number of things we can do to help.

Sharing activities

Most people make friends with those who share their interests and values (e.g. members of the same political party, football team, work colleagues, fellow students). Therefore, helping people to engage in activities or join groups/clubs/religious communities in which they might meet like-minded people can be important. However, it may also be useful to help people think about ways of moving beyond simple shared activity by taking steps to extend relationships outwith the boundaries of the activity. This might include, for example, going out for a drink after work/college/the football match, or engaging in other social activities such as going to the cinema, or inviting someone round for coffee.

Using Internet chat lines and e-groups

Some people may find it difficult to go out and make contact with people. Perhaps they live in a geographically isolated place or have problems that make socialising difficult. With the birth of the Internet and the increasing availability of computers, it is becoming more common for people to make contact with each other via internet e-groups and chat lines. Some of these enable people with similar interests to contact each other. Some enable people to regain contact with people they have known in the past: for example,

Friends Reunited enables people to get in touch with old school friends. Others – such as the Uksurvivors e-group – specifically enable people who have experienced mental health problems to make contact with, and gain support from, each other.

'Lonely hearts' columns

'Lonely hearts' columns and dating agencies provide many people – whether or not they have mental health problems – with the opportunity to meet others with a view to friendship or more intimate relationships. Perhaps mental health workers may help people to respond to personal adverts in local papers or listings magazines, or to place advertisements of their own. In doing this it is important to remind people of basic safety precautions (such as not initially meeting people at home or in a secluded place).

'Befriending'

'Befriending' can help to bring together a volunteer 'befriender' and an isolated service-user, both of whom are interested in increasing their social contacts and sharing activities.

Facilitating contact between people who have mental health problems

Friendships and relationships with people who have experienced similar difficulties can be very important. Mental health workers may be able to promote such relationships in a number of ways:

◆ Facilitating access to shared activities (e.g. fishing trips, opportunities to go to concerts, clubs, etc.) for small groups of people who share common interests

◆ Helping people to join self-help groups and user/survivor organisations

◆ Offering 'buddy' schemes in which people with mental health problems can 'befriend' others with similar difficulties

◆ Offering opportunities for people to seek others with similar interests and concerns (e.g. one service provided a notice-board on which people could post notices asking if there was anyone who fancied going to the pictures, or the pub, etc.).

We all do much to promote inclusion on a daily basis. We might, for example, ask a new neighbour round for coffee and tell him/her about good places to go in the local area, or we might invite a new pupil at our child's school round for tea. We might talk through how a colleague could tackle a difficult work situation they face. We might help a friend who is trying to resolve difficulties in his/her marriage. Within mental health services many practitioners already help people to do a great many things that they want to do, but there exists little to guide these endeavours. While extensive research exists on the relative merits of different therapeutic approaches, and there is an emerging literature on ways of helping people to access employment and education, there is little concerning ways of helping people to access other social and leisure opportunities. Indeed, the different methods that might be adopted have rarely been itemised, leaving mental health workers reliant solely on their own experience and on the ideas of others with whom they have worked. We have tried to go some way towards providing such an inventory in Chapter 11. In so doing we are indebted to the work of Peter Bates in compiling an *A–Z of Socially Inclusive Strategies* (unpublished, 2002).

11

Some strategies for promoting inclusion

INTRODUCTION

Any help that mental health workers provide to enable people to access the things they want to do must be tailored to their individual needs and preferences, and to the demands of the situation. The strategies that we describe in this chapter do not constitute a 'blueprint' for inclusion. Nor can we treat them as items on a menu from which a selection can be made. It is likely to be necessary to use a number of different approaches, and to tailor each to the person's unique circumstances. We do not pretend to offer a comprehensive account of all possible approaches, but hope that the reader will use the material we present creatively to develop, with the people whom they are assisting, new and different solutions.

PROVIDING INFORMATION ABOUT OPPORTUNITIES IN THE LOCAL AREA

Information is an essential prerequisite for access: if you do not know what is available, you cannot avail yourself of it. Going into an unfamiliar situation is scary for most people. Even a simple thing like going into a new café can present problems: do you sit down and wait for someone to take your order, or do you order at the counter? When you have ordered, do you stand and wait for your food, or sit down and wait for someone to bring it? When you have finished, do you ask for a bill and pay the waiter, or go to the till and pay?

Most things are easier if we know what is expected of us in advance. Mental health workers can help people to get this information in a number of ways:

◆ Describe what the activity is like, what it offers, and what the person would have to do to use it. Perhaps it may be possible to show them pictures or brochures.

◆ Arrange for the person to meet someone from the facility so that they can explain what to do. For example, ask the supervisor at the local supermarket to describe what working in the shop involves, or ask the Imam to explain what the local mosque offers.

◆ Help the person to make contact with someone who is already using the facility. Perhaps there are other service-users that the person could talk to? Perhaps they have friends or relatives who could help?

PROVIDING AN INVENTORY OF WHAT PEOPLE DO WHEN ENGAGING IN AN ACTIVITY

Making an inventory of what people do when engaging in an activity does not simply involve looking at written guidelines or guessing what people probably do. There can be a big difference between the formal expectations of a college course, workplace, sports club or church, and what people actually do. For example, at the bingo hall, there are likely to be 'regulars' who always sit in particular seats, so if you want to 'fit in' it is best to sit somewhere else. At the swimming baths, perhaps people leave their towels in the locker rather than taking them through to the pool with them. Perhaps women never go in to 'The George' pub on their own, and there's never anyone over about 30 in 'The Dragon'. At work, perhaps colleagues stop to say hello to the doorman on the way in, the supervisor always has his/her cup of tea first, and if the manager's door is closed it means he/she does not want to be disturbed. Knowledge of these 'unwritten rules' can make all the difference to whether a person is accepted or not.

Even where formal guidelines do exist, they often tell you little about what is really expected. For example, at the college, it may say that all assignments have to be in on time. In reality, people may regularly ask the tutor for an extension. At work, 'job descriptions' and 'terms and conditions of employment' rarely tell you what you are actually expected to do. In order to help people with mental health problems prepare for employment it is often useful to go and watch people at work. This has been an important component of the work of the 'job coach' (see below) and has been used to good effect in a number of supported employment programmes like that described by Perkins et al (2001b). An employment support worker 'shadowed' someone already doing the job and put the tasks together into a manual that was used both in induction and as a reference guide for the supported employee when he/she was unsure what to do. These manuals proved so useful that managers gave them to new recruits who did not have mental health problems.

In finding out what people really do there is no substitute for actually going and having a look. The task of compiling an inventory of what people do does not have to be restricted to the mental health worker: service-users can go and see for themselves. This involvement can alert them to the need to watch what others do and then follow suit. The axiom 'When in Rome do as the Romans do', is important for all of us.

PLANNING AND TARGET SETTING

Planning and target-setting helps people to think about their ambitions and plan the interim goals on the way to achieving them. Most people's ambitions cannot be achieved immediately. We cannot just decide to 'get married and have children' or 'become a nurse'. Instead, we need to look at what is required to achieve the ambition and plan how to move towards it. For example, if we want to 'get married and have children' we first have to find a mate, and this means going to places where we might meet someone we can get on with. This may involve thinking about our likes and dislikes and where we might meet someone who shares them. For example, a committed Labour Party supporter might be likely to meet kindred spirits by joining the local party, while someone with particular religious beliefs might find like-minded people at the local church. Next, we need to think about how we can get to know the people we meet better; perhaps we can ask if they would like to go out for a drink after the meeting. If someone wants to be a nurse, he/she first needs to look at what extra qualifications and experience is needed for eligibility for a training course.

The critical part of this process is to ensure that we help the client to break down the 'journey' into manageable steps. However, in doing this three things are important.

First, people must be able to see that they are achieving something that matters to them at each stage. It is very easy to give up if you do not think you are getting anywhere. Some people feel that they are achieving more if they do something they really want to do, but require assistance to do it (e.g. going to an ordinary course at the local college with someone to help them). Others experience a greater sense of achievement when they can reach an intermediate aim unaided (e.g. going to a specialist class for people with mental health problems).

Second, it is as important to pay as much attention to progression as to starting the journey in the first place. It is very easy for both the mental health worker and the person they are assisting to lose sight of the eventual aim. For example, if a person needs to gain qualifications in order to get a job he/she wants, then the first step may be going to college. In order to prevent this from becoming an end in itself, it is important to review progress, plan the next course, help them to get relevant 'work experience', and so forth.

Third, people's goals change. As we do things, we see different possibilities and we may want to change direction. Therefore, it is important, from time to time, to help people review where they wish to go – and accept that people may change course many times before they find something they want to do.

PRACTICE

Practice helps people to rehearse what they are going to do until they feel comfortable doing it. When faced with things that we are wary about, many of us find it useful to practice what we might say or do beforehand. Personally speaking, we have both practiced talks that we are going to give at conferences, and answers we might give in job interviews – and tried on different outfits in order to decide which one to wear on the big day! It can be helpful for a person to practice what he/she will say when, for example, he/she goes to register for a college course, join the library, or invite someone out for a drink.

With practice, confidence and skills improve, though some people get very dispirited when they do not get something right first time. It is important that both practitioners and the people whom they are helping remember that it took a great deal of practice for all of us to do the things that we now take for granted – speaking, walking, cooking, reading. In writing this book we rehearsed lots of different ways of organising the material and saying the things we wanted to say before we arrived at the version that you are reading now.

It is important for mental health workers to remember that people may have to do the same thing over and over again before they feel comfortable doing it. If, for example, a person has not been out on his/her own for some time, he/she is likely to feel apprehensive. Practitioners may be tempted to take a person to a variety of different destinations in helping him/her to go out again, but this may not always be the best approach. In order to gain the confidence that comes with familiarity, some people find it easier to go to the same place (the same café, or shop, or park) a number of times until they feel at ease before moving on to different places.

It is easy for people's skills to get 'rusty' during periods when they are unable to engage in their usual activities; practice can help people maintain competencies. For example, opportunities to practice work, study, leisure and domestic skills during an in-patient admission can help to maintain these abilities, enabling that person to use a computer, do some typing, read, cook their own meals, go jogging, etc.

SKILLS DEVELOPMENT

A variety of techniques can be used to help people develop the skills they need in order to do the things they want to do. Skills-training approaches have long been popular in helping people to develop the repertoire of competencies they need in order to live independently (see Anthony 1977, 1994, Antony et al 1984). Such approaches start by identifying the skills involved in performing the activity, whether it be filling out an application form, making a cup of tea, or going to the pub. The second stage involves looking at the person's performance and assessing where problems exist. Finally, on the basis of this analysis, steps are taken systematically to help a person to develop the competencies they need. There are various strategies that can be adopted (see, for example, Barker 1982), most commonly:

◆ Instruction: this involves telling the person how to do what he/she needs to do.

◆ Prompting: this means reminding the person what to do next.

◆ Modelling: this involves watching how someone else does something and then copying him/her. In this context, the characteristics of the model are important. First, 'coping' models are more effective than 'mastery' models. Someone who is only just able to do the task (i.e. appears to be rather anxious or has some difficulty) is likely to be a more effective model than someone who makes it all look very easy. Second, we are more likely to acquire skills from someone whom we perceive as similar to ourselves. In a mental health context, this means that people with mental health problems are likely to be more effective models than more distant staff members or other experts.

◆ Guided practice: this means doing something alongside someone and guiding him/her through what he/she needs to do.

◆ Feedback: this involves reviewing what the person has done, making a point of emphasising the parts they have done well, the progress they have made, as well as the areas that still need more work.

In skills training, a great deal has been written about 'contingency management' and 'schedules of reinforcement'. However, it is our experience that helping people to achieve something they want to do is reinforcing in itself: they feel good about what they have managed to do, so additional 'reinforcement' is unnecessary. The critical issue is whether we are helping people to do the things they wish to do or the things we think they ought to do. Promoting inclusion is not about doing things to people, but about helping them to explore what they want to do themselves. It may, however, be necessary to help people see what they have achieved. If you find it difficult to do something that others seem to take in their stride, then you may be tempted to undervalue what you have accomplished. For example, as one person told us:

When I first went on the underground I felt great – as if I'd really done something. Then I thought 'What's the big deal, I'm an adult, anyone can go on the train?'. Then I realised that while it might not be a big deal for most people, I have been in hospital for over 20 years and going on the tube is a big deal for me, and I managed it. That's something to be proud of. (cited in Perkins & Repper 1996)

A number of studies have demonstrated that it is better to learn how to do something in the situation in which you will normally do it. There can be problems in generalising from one situation to another (Shepherd 1977, 1978). So if you want to learn how to cook, it is better to do so in your own kitchen. If you want to learn how to do a job, it is better to do so in the job than in a sheltered workshop first (Bond et al 1997, 2001). For example, 'job coaches' have proved helpful for some people: someone first learns the job himself/herself and then teaches you when you start work and supports you until you can manage on your own.

It is also important to ensure that the training process does not make people feel belittled or infantilised. They are unlikely to persist in learning how to do something if the training process makes them feel stupid. Similarly, while some people find the presence of a 'job coach' helpful, others find that it singles them out as different and makes them look incompetent (see Perkins et al 2001a). Some prefer to receive assistance outside the work, college or social/leisure setting (e.g. on the end of a telephone perhaps, or by meeting up afterwards to review the day) rather than having someone with them.

Finally, simply having the skills is not enough. Some people need ongoing support to do the things they want to do. This does not mean that they, or the mental health workers, have 'failed', merely that the service-users need a different sort of help. Research on supporting people with mental health problems in open employment clearly indicates that the presence of support without limit of time is very important in helping many people to retain work (Bond et al 1997, 2001, Evans & Repper 1998).

GRADED EXPOSURE

'Graded exposure' helps people to overcome fears that stop them doing what they want to do. If a person wants to do something, but is anxious about doing it, then graded exposure may be useful. This involves helping the person to develop a hierarchy of the things that scare them in relation to an activity. Most of us feel less anxious when we are with someone we trust than when we are on our own. Therefore, when thinking about the hierarchy of fears, it is important to think about both the tasks involved and the support available. For example, if a person wants to go to a pub he/she may feel less anxious when he/she is with someone, when the pub is not crowded, and when he/she does not have to go to the bar and buy drinks. Their 'fear hier-archy' may therefore be as follows (the least-feared situation being shown first):

◆ going to an uncrowded pub with someone else who buys the drinks
◆ going to an uncrowded pub with someone else and going to the bar with him/her to buy the drinks
◆ going to an uncrowded pub with someone else and going to the bar alone to buy the drinks
◆ going to an uncrowded pub alone but meeting someone else there
◆ going to an uncrowded pub alone and buying a drink
◆ going to a crowded pub with someone else who buys the drinks
◆ going to a crowded pub with someone else and going to the bar with him/her to buy the drinks
◆ going to a crowded pub with someone else and going to the bar alone to buy the drinks
◆ going to a crowded pub alone but meeting someone else there
◆ going to a crowded pub alone and buying a drink

Graded exposure would involve starting with the least anxiety-provoking situation and gradually moving to the more anxiety-provoking ones as the person's confidence increases.

In using graded exposure it is important that the mental health worker tailors the approach to the individual's preferences. Different aspects of the same situation cause anxiety to different people. People wish to progress through the things that scare them in various ways. Some may wish to 'get it all over at once' and start with the most scary situation (sometimes called 'flooding'). Others may wish to start in the middle of the list rather than at the bottom. Some may find that after they have mastered the first step they want to jump to the middle or the top of the list. Others may wish to insert different steps they had not originally thought of. Some may decide to stop at a particular stage. For example, someone might decide that he/she would never want to go to a pub on his/her own and is content with being able to go with friends. Some may have a go, decide it is not worth the effort, and give up completely!

It is, however, important that at each stage, the person feels he/she has achieved something. In their desire to help people to 'be independent', some mental health workers set great store by people doing things unaided. So, in helping them to go to the pub, they may start by suggesting that the person simply goes to the pub and then walks away, then steps through the door and leaves immediately, then sits down for a few minutes but does not buy a drink, and so forth. Using this method, it will be some time before the person actually gets a drink and they may become dispirited and give up ('What's the point, I'm not getting anywhere'.) It is generally preferable to provide the person with the help they need to achieve something that he/she finds meaningful from the start, and then gradually withdraw this support. In the hierarchy described above, the person actually gets to go out for a drink from the start – but with someone they trust and with this person going to the bar for them.

GRADED RETURN

'Graded return' is a return to activities following a period of absence caused by relapse and/or hospital admission. It is preferable to help a person to retain the roles that he/she already has, rather than waiting until these have been lost and trying to rebuild them. A crisis often prevents a person from doing the things that he/she usually does; resuming them once the crisis has passed can be problematic. Going back to work, meeting up with friends, or going back to the sports club can be very difficult: how do you explain why you have been away? It is even harder if, because of the crisis, you have behaved in uncharacteristic ways. Facing people again after you have let them down, or done things that you feel embarrassed about, can be extremely tricky. If the person does not go back as soon as he/she can, however, then it may be impossible to go back at all. Mental health workers – as well as friends and relatives – can ease the return.

While the person is still in hospital – or 'out of circulation' – mental health workers can support him/her in explaining to friends, managers, colleagues, fellow students and others why he/she is absent. Perhaps the person can be helped to write a letter explaining that he/she is ill and will be back as soon as possible, or, with his/her permission, call and explain what has happened on his/her behalf or ask a friend or relative to do so.

Once the crisis has begun to abate, the practitioner can help the person to resume some activities even while he/she is still in hospital. Perhaps arrangements can be made for friends to visit or for the person to start going to church; perhaps the practitioner can get some work from the person's manager to help him/her to begin to catch up with what has been missed. It is unlikely that the person will feel able to take up all the usual activities immediately, but it is important to begin the process in a graded way as soon as possible: the longer he/she is away the more difficult it is to go back. A number of strategies can facilitate this:

◆ Help the person to decide what they want to say to people about why they have been absent.
◆ Make plans for initial contacts with managers, colleagues, people from the faith community, friends, tutors, etc.
◆ Provide practical assistance (transport, going with the person, etc.).

◆ Be available to provide encouragement and assist with difficulties that arise.

◆ Help the person and others involved to plan a graded return. Each individual will have different preferences, but a graded plan for returning to college might involve:

- an initial meeting with the tutor to make plans
- taking some work home to catch up
- going in to meet fellow students socially (e.g. having a cup of coffee with them at break-time)
- starting to go to one or two classes initially and then gradually building up attendance
- help to get to college (continued until the person feels able to get there unaided)
- being available on the telephone so that the person can call if he/she has problems
- calling or meeting the person after the first day to review how things have gone and make plans for the next day (and thereafter, until the person no longer needs the support)
- gradually reducing the support provided as the person's confidence increases
- making plans for, and providing, ongoing support
- making plans for how to deal with future crises should they arise.

Many similar elements might also be useful in helping the person to resume work, contact with friends and engagement in other social activities.

'JUST VISITING'

Just visiting a place beforehand is a way of becoming familiar with how to get there and what to expect. It is usually easier to do something when you know what it is like. Therefore, it can be helpful just to go and have a look before 'taking the plunge'. For example, if you want to go to the swimming pool, it may be helpful to work out which bus to use, where to catch it and, where to get off, and to have a look at the place before actually going for a swim. Perhaps it would be helpful to go into the reception area, see what people are doing, and pick up a leaflet about opening times, etc.

'TIME-LIMITED EXPERIENCE'

Time-limited experience is a way of trying something out before deciding whether you want to do it. Work experience is probably the most widely used example of this type of approach. It involves working somewhere for a few weeks to find out what it involves before deciding whether to apply for a job.

In this instance, there is the added advantage that the employer gets to see what the person can do, which may enhance his/her chance of getting a job there, or at least furnish him/her with a reference. Although there are formal 'work-experience' schemes organised by the Employment Service and various other specialist agencies, in our experience it is also possible to negotiate work experience on a more informal basis. For example, one young man wanted to work in a health-food shop, so the mental health worker went to a local health-food shop with him and helped him to ask if he could work there for one or two days a week to get some experience. The young man decided that he liked the work, but did not feel able to work full time, so after he had shown what he could do, he was offered a paid 'Saturday Job'. We have also known a number of people who have preferred to set up such work-experience placements for themselves or with the help of their relatives or friends.

In addition, some community facilities (colleges, sports centres, etc.) organise 'taster sessions' or 'open days' when people can go and find out what is on offer. It may also be possible to negotiate for a person to visit on a less formal basis.

PROVIDING TRANSPORT

Providing transport can help a person to get to an activity. Many people find travelling difficult and this can act as a major barrier to doing the things they want to do. Even if the person is able to use public transport, it may be just too daunting to have to undertake both a complicated journey and a new activity all at the same time. In such instances, access can be facilitated by arranging transport to take the person to the sports centre, workplace, library, cinema or whatever. A small budget for taxis, or volunteer drivers, can be enormously helpful in facilitating access and if these are not available then the 'taxi-service' role of the mental health worker should not be overlooked.

'DOING WITH'

It is often easier to go to a strange place or start something new if you can do it with someone else. Mental health workers have long taken the role of escort – helping people to go to all manner of places and do all manner of things. While this has undoubtedly helped a large number of people, it is important that the way in which the support is provided does not attract negative attention. When we lead someone along by the hand, give them instructions, tell them what to do and what not to do, and speak for the person, it is often all too obvious that he/she is a patient being escorted by a member of staff. We should aim to be as unobtrusive as possible, i.e. to 'pass' as the person's friend or relative rather than their 'helper'.

There are many people other than staff members who may more appropriately accompany the person. Many people would prefer to do things with friends or relatives than with staff members. If friends and relatives are not available, volunteers or 'befrienders' might be. Perhaps there is another member of the church, or sports club, or a colleague who might be happy to help the person? Most importantly, people with mental health problems can, and do, help each other. For example, we know one man who goes to a computer course with another service-user who would not have been able to go alone. Another young man regularly accompanies a fellow resident in his hostel (an older woman who uses a wheelchair) to the shops, pub and betting shop.

SUBSIDY

Helping to meet the costs of activities is important. Poverty greatly limits inclusion: almost every activity requires some form of expenditure that is often beyond the slender means of people who live on state benefits. Giving people the money they need can make all the difference in helping them to do the things they want to do: go to the cinema; get the bus to visit a friend; register for a college course; get lunch in the canteen; go out for a meal with other students; or put money in the collection at the church service.

It is also important to explore other sources of subsidy, e.g. grants to buy a computer or for study, reduced rates at colleges, sports and leisure facilities for people who are unemployed, bus passes and reduced entry fees for disabled people, and so forth. Similarly, there are sometimes Employment Service schemes that subsidise employers who take on disabled people, or pay for any adjustments or support they need in order to access work.

SPECIAL GROUPS WITHIN ORDINARY SETTINGS

Sometimes people feel more confident in starting a new activity if, at least initially, they are with others who have similar difficulties. Such groups may be provided either by mental health workers or by people in the situation. Some examples we have encountered include the following:

◆ Groups organised at the local sports centre by sports therapists to introduce people with mental health problems to the facilities

◆ Special classes for people with mental health problems in colleges (organised by mental heath workers and/or college staff) to enable them to get used to study and explore the opportunities available

◆ Work crews, where an employment project contracts to provide a service to a business (for example, a contract to deliver cleaning, gardening or internal mail) and a group of people with mental health problems go to the business to do the work assisted by a mental health worker.

If people are to be able to move from the special, segregated group to use the facility alongside other non-disabled participants, then a graded plan can be helpful. For example, students could be encouraged to register for other non-segregated courses in the college while at the same time continuing to receive support from the special course until they no longer need it.

STAFF FROM DIFFERENT COMMUNITY FACILITIES/GROUPS COMING INTO MENTAL HEALTH SERVICES

Sometimes people do not feel sufficiently confident to use ordinary facilities, or perhaps there are legal restrictions that prevent them from doing so. It may therefore be necessary to arrange for people from these organisations to come into the mental health services. We know of the following examples:

◆ tutors from local colleges coming in to run classes
◆ musicians from a local music project running music sessions
◆ members of faith communities visiting people in hospitals and secure units
◆ contract work from external agencies being brought in to mental health facilities (e.g. we have seen people in a high-secure hospital typesetting information booklets for a local authority, and detained patients in a psychiatric service assembling 'poppies' for 'poppy day', and proofreading manuscripts and doing various administrative jobs for local businesses).

However, if people are really to have access to the range of ordinary opportunities available in the community, it is important that such initiatives are seen as 'a step on the way' rather than an end in themselves. People can be assisted to take courses at the local college, to go down to the music project, to join in church activities, and to access ordinary jobs in integrated settings as soon as possible.

MENTORING

Mentoring is a way of obtaining support from someone engaged in the activity. Often we can learn a great deal about what an activity involves and how we might do it from someone who is already doing it. Their guidance can greatly assist us in getting the job or the place on a course that we want, or in joining the local swimming club or political group. When we start the activity, having someone to show us the ropes can also be enormously helpful.

ADAPTATION AND ADJUSTMENT ON THE PART OF THE PROVIDER

Changes to the physical or social environment or the expectations of the person may be necessary to facilitate access. British Disability Discrimination legislation not only outlaws discrimination against disabled people – explicitly including people with mental health problems – but also requires that employers and the providers of education, goods and services make 'reasonable adjustments' to ensure that the disabled person can access the opportunities they offer. Often such 'adjustments' are considered only in terms of the modifications to the physical environment that people with mobility or sensory impairments might need, e.g. lowered desks, ramps, hearing loops and so forth. However, there is an equal obligation to make 'reasonable adjustments' to facilitate access by people with mental health problems.

In the context of adjustments, it is important to remember that social roles (e.g. worker, father, friend) are not defined by a fixed set of expectations. Roles are relational, i.e. negotiated between the people involved (Shepherd 1984, Perkins & Repper 1996). There is no set of skills that defines a worker or a father. The role of father differs from family to family and can change over time. Different people doing the same job will do it differently, bringing different skills and personal attributes to the tasks involved. Roles can be negotiated and renegotiated to accommodate mental health difficulties. This might mean working with families, social networks, employers and college tutors to renegotiate roles and their associated expectations. For example, a student may generally be expected to complete his/her studies within a given period of time, but this can be difficult if there are absences because of mental health problems. In order for a person to access the course, expectations might have to be adjusted, e.g. it might take four years to do what is usually a two-year course, or the student might study at home rather than always having to go into college.

Similarly, much work with families might usefully be understood in terms of changing roles and expectations. One young man with whom we worked left university because of his mental health problems. This forced a renegotiation of roles: a young man who had left home and was becoming independent returned to dependence on his parents. Initially, his role became one of a young child, and his parents did almost everything for him and made decisions on his behalf. Clearly, this did not allow him to develop and use his skills, so the family were helped to negotiate the expectations they had of each other once again. The young man began to take on the role of helping his aging parents: doing the garden, decorating, and going shopping for them. He also began to do voluntary work at the local charity shop. So from having the role of a young child he was able to make an important contribution to family life and become a valued voluntary worker.

A key role of the mental health worker is to help people to identify what adjustments they might need and, where necessary, to help them to negotiate these. Sometimes it may be necessary for employers/providers to be gently reminded of their legal obligations. [The Disability Rights Commission Helpline (Tel.: 08457 622633. Textphone: 08457 62644) can be useful, both for people with mental health problems and for mental health practitioners, in providing advice and assistance in this area.] The identification of adjustments that people with mental health problems might need is still in its infancy. At the time of writing, consideration of 'reasonable adjustments' for people with mental health problems is probably most developed in the field of employment (see, for example, Boston Center for Psychiatric Rehabilitation 2002). Adaptations that may be helpful in employment include the following:

◆ Good induction into the job may be important. Many 'job descriptions' are very vague and the resulting uncertainty can be very anxiety-provoking, thus aggravating the person's difficulties.

◆ It can be helpful to have a workplace mentor (see above) who can take the new employee under his/her wing.

◆ Increased supervision and feedback may be necessary so that the person knows how well he/she is doing and which areas require development.

◆ Someone whom the person can ask if he/she is unsure of what to do, without fear of being seen as incompetent, can be helpful.

◆ Time off for regular mental health or therapy appointments may be required. Sometimes schedules can be reorganised so that the person does not miss work time: shifts can be arranged around the person's commitments, or lost time can be made up for by starting earlier or finishing later.

◆ Access to a telephone may be useful so that the person can call a friend or support worker if he/she is having problems.

◆ Flexible working hours (as in 'flexi-time') may be useful if, for example, the person finds it difficult to travel in crowded rush-hour buses. Working later shifts if the person finds the mornings difficult, or the possibility of part-time working, or regular breaks, are other useful options.

◆ Provision for a support worker to help the person do the job might be helpful (although this can attract negative attention to the person and often help is better offered off-site; see Perkins et al 2001b).

◆ Adjustments in the physical environment, such as having a desk somewhere quiet to avoid distractions, may help some people.

It may be difficult for a person to ask for adjustments. He/she may fear that the employer will think him/her unable to do the job. It may be useful for mental health workers to help people think about how they can ask for what they need, or to help them to negotiate their requirements. Often the adjustments that people require are easily achieved, but there is no set formula: adaptations must be tailored around the individual concerned. Many of the adjustments listed above may improve the performance of any employee: things like good induction, regular supervision and appraisal, mentoring for new staff, and an environment where people can ask if they are unsure what to do are likely to improve the work performance of anyone. Some adjustments may be required by other employees, not just those with mental health problems. For example, someone who has caring responsibilities or is attending a college course may require flexible working arrangements, and anyone who is returning to work after a long period (because of unemployment, caring for children, or physical health problems) might require extra supervision and support to build up his/her confidence.

It is also important not to assume that because a person has mental health problems he/she will automatically need special adjustments. Many people are able to engage in a range of activities and get the support they need from family, friends or mental health workers. Perkins et al (2001b) described the range of different types of support that people using one supported employment programme required. Most involved help, outside the workplace: filling in application forms, preparing for interview, sorting out benefits, providing encouragement, or resolving difficulties within or outwith work that might interfere with the ability to do the job. These may all be 'adjustments' on the part of mental health workers rather than employers.

Many of the adjustments that facilitate access to work can also facilitate access to other social, educational and leisure opportunities. Perhaps a person needs to 'sit on the sidelines' for a while rather than be encouraged to join in from the start. Perhaps he/she needs to leave the activity early or take breaks. Activities that operate in the afternoon or evening may be easier than those in the morning. Modular courses that allow someone to take breaks if he/she has problems can be helpful. A great deal will depend on the ingenuity of the people involved, including mental health workers, people with mental health problems, employers and other providers.

SELF-ADJUSTMENT/ADAPTATION

People can be helped to work out adjustments they can make themselves to facilitate access. Many people with mental health problems do not need to rely on the employers, colleges or providers of leisure/social activities to make adjustments. Unbeknown to the employers (or other providers), many people make their own adjustments to ensure that they can do the things they want to do. Leete (1989) (see Chapter 10) offers a number of ways in which she has done this at work. One woman we know, who worked as a health-care assistant in a psychiatric ward, experienced limited periods of time when she found it difficult to interact with other staff members and residents. At such times, she offered to check the stock room or file notes. As these were unpopular jobs, her offers were invariably accepted; no one knew they were making 'adjustments'. Another man found that, from time to time, his 'voices' got particularly bad and he just had to talk back to them, but he was worried what other people would think if he did this at the church 'social'. The solution he worked out was to go to the toilet and speak to them in private.

In helping someone to think about the adjustments they might make, a number of considerations are helpful:

◆ It is important to tailor the coping strategy to the particular situation, e.g. going to the toilet may be feasible at church, but is not a solution to demanding 'voices' on the bus.

◆ If a mental health worker is to be of assistance in working out ways of coping with symptoms, they must know what is possible in that situation, i.e. go and find out for themselves.

◆ Mental health workers should not assume they are the font of all wisdom:

– often it is better to help people to think through what has worked in other situations, or explore their own ideas about ways of coping, rather than telling them what to do

– other people who have coped with similar symptoms or problems are often in a better position to advise.

DELIBERATELY INTEGRATED GROUPS

The creation of specific settings in which people with mental health problems and those who do not experience such difficulties can do things together can be helpful. This does not involve recruiting people who do not have mental health problems to assist those who have such difficulties. Instead it involves providing a forum where people with and without mental health problems can meet as equals. For example, in a work context, a 'social firm' is a fully commercial enterprise that pays the going rate for the job, but in which a proportion of the workforce (usually at least 25%) comprises people who have mental health difficulties (Grove et al 1997).

HELP AND SUPPORT WHEN DIFFICULTIES ARISE

Many people with mental health problems are able to engage, unaided, in a range of activities most of the time. However, the fluctuating nature of mental health problems means that there may be times when people have difficulties. It is very easy for a person to 'drop out' at such times unless support is readily available. In providing sensitive and effective support, a number of factors may be important:

◆ The individual's preferences: people like to receive assistance in different ways, so it is wise to ask. Many people do not want to need assistance, and feel inadequate if they are unable to do things unaided; therefore it may be important to offer assistance in an unobtrusive fashion. If, for example, someone is having difficulty getting to an activity, help could be offered in an 'up-front' way ('I can see you are having difficulties, would you like me to give you a lift?') or less obtrusively ('I've got to go into town next Tuesday and I'll be going past your house – would you like a lift?').

◆ Assistance must be available at the time the person needs it: having to wait for a weekly or monthly appointment may be too late. In this context, telephone support may be useful (see Perkins et al 2001b).

◆ Preference should be given to 'natural supports' that already exist in the setting. Some employers have counselling or 'employee-assistance' programmes, and some colleges have student support services. Is it possible for the person to ask the help of colleagues or other participants (e.g. by saying that he/she is not feeling 'too good today') so that others do not expect too much of them?

◆ The help should be provided in a way that does not disrupt the activity or draw negative attention to the person. An older female mental health worker can, for example, look very out of place in an activity for young men.

SELF-HELP GROUPS

People in a similar position are often well placed to help each other. Sometimes this is achieved in an informal way whereby people simply help each other out; at other times, formal 'support groups' can be helpful.

Some self-help groups are available to everyone involved in the setting whether or not they have mental health problems (e.g. support groups for colleagues at work, or for students at college). By enabling a person with mental health problems to access such support arrangements, he/she may see that everyone is experiencing similar stresses and strains. At other times, people with mental health problems might benefit from sharing experiences that are particularly associated with their difficulties. These groups may fall into different categories:

◆ Generic groups allow people engaged in a wide range of pursuits and activities, or with a broad spectrum of interests, to share experience.

◆ Some groups are focused on specific subsets of people with common concerns, e.g. a mental health group for women, or for people from minority ethnic groups, or a 'hearing voices' group.

◆ Other groups are organised around shared interests, as is the case with Survivors' Poetry and a range of campaigning and political action groups.

◆ Certain groups are specifically tailored to people involved in a particular activity, such as those organised for employees or students with mental health problems.

Support groups may be open (anyone can join in) or closed (restricted to a named group of people). They may be facilitated – either by one of the group members in a 'self-help' arrangement' or by an 'external' facilitator or support worker. Different models will undoubtedly suit different people and situations. However, there is a danger that if the group is facilitated by someone who is regarded as an 'expert' then group members will turn to them for advice, rather than recognising their own 'expertise of experience'.

SELECTING AN APPROPRIATE STRATEGY FOR WORKING WITH INDIVIDUALS

There are many ways in which we might facilitate inclusion, and it is important to select the appropriate strategy for each individual and situation.

Individual acceptability.

What sort of help does the person want? One person may not feel safe unless a mental health worker is present, while another would not wish to 'be seen dead' with a member of staff. As in other areas, we need to move beyond a 'professional knows best' approach and accept that people are able to decide for themselves what sort of help they want. It may be helpful for the mental health worker to describe the different possible ways in which support could be provided.

Social acceptability

Different approaches to helping a person may be more or less obvious to others and draw more or less negative attention to the person who is receiving the help. In general, help should minimise the negative attention that it attracts. While individuals differ in their preferences, ordinary resources that are available to everyone in the community are generally more socially acceptable than specialist mental health resources. Assistance from peers, friends and relatives is generally more socially acceptable than help from a mental health practitioner.

Issues of control

Most people do not want to need help, but assistance is generally more acceptable when it is under the control of the person who is receiving it, i.e. when the person can determine what help is received, who provides it, and how, when and where it is provided.

Help received in the past

What has been tried before and to what effect? Unless the person and his/her circumstances have changed markedly, what worked in the past is probably worth trying again. What did not work is best avoided. The person who is on the receiving end is usually in the best position to tell us what has worked for him/her.

The amount of support a person needs

Some people need more support than others. While one person needs only to know what is available in order to decide what to do, others may need more intense help to achieve their goals.

The amount of support available

Resource constraints are an ever-present reality and it is important that the person who is deciding what sort of help he/she wants is aware of these constraints; unrealisable 'wish lists' are of no value to anyone. However, it is important to remember that mental health resources do not define the limits of support available. There are many sources of assistance to be found outside such services: advice centres, help lines, support groups, assistance from friends, relatives or volunteers, etc. A bit of lateral thinking can go a long way!

The type of expertise required

Mental health workers may have expertise in mental health issues, but this is rarely the only type of expertise required to help people to do the things they want to do in the world outside mental health services. If you want a job, you need employment expertise, if you want to go to college, educational expertise is required, and if you want to make sure you get all the benefits you are entitled to, welfare-rights expertise is of the essence. If people with mental health problems are to have access to the best help available then mental health practitioners should facilitate access to specialist sources of assistance rather than trying to take on everything themselves.

The person's existing contacts and resources

Many people who use mental health services already have friends, relatives and contacts who can assist them to do the things they want to do.

The research evidence on effectiveness

A body of research is beginning to accumulate on the effectiveness of different types of help and support. For example, research into the effectiveness of skills training strongly indicates that skills should be taught in the environment in which they will be used. Skills learned in one environment do not 'translate' well to other settings (Shepherd 1977, 1978, Scott et al 1984, Anthony et al 1984, Appelo et al 1992, Ekdawi & Conning 1994).

A number of research studies on access to employment have demonstrated that the type of support offered is a more important determinant of success than are psychiatric problems and symptoms (Secker & Membury 2000, Secker et al 2001). The sheltered workshops that have been so popular in the UK are intended to help people to develop the skills, confidence and work routines they need in order to move on to open employment. However, research suggests that they are not effective in these efforts (Pozner et al 1996): very few people ever move on to open employment. Instead, research clearly demonstrates that six key factors are important to the success of programmes designed to help people to gain and sustain open employment (Bond et al 1997, 2001, Crowther et al 2001):

◆ The primary goal should be one of permanent employment in integrated settings, i.e. 'real work'.

◆ Rapid job search and minimal pre-vocational training, i.e. 'place–train' models (in which a person is helped to get a job and is then trained on the job), are more effective than the more conventional 'train–place' approaches in which people are first taught a range of work skills in a sheltered setting and then assisted to find a job.

◆ Clinical treatment should be integrated with vocational rehabilitation. Vocational support should be an integral part of the work of the mental health team: all staff members need a vocational orientation, and specialist vocational expertise should be available to the team.

◆ Attention should be given to the preferences of the user. People are more likely to stick at a job they want than to the one the clinicians think appropriate.

◆ Assessment should continue after employment. Getting into work is not an end in itself but part of an ongoing process of helping the person to develop and move on, and adjusting the support they need.

◆ Time-unlimited support and workplace intervention are needed to help the person sustain his/her employment.

Similar principles are likely to be equally important in helping people to access education (c.f. Unger et al 1991, Wertheimer 1997), but, in addition, flexible course design (e.g. modular courses which allow students to drop in and out, and distance-learning approaches) appears to be beneficial for some people.

Traditional approaches to facilitating access for people who have mental health problems have tended to focus solely on developing people's competencies. While personal growth and development are important in helping people to rebuild their lives, they are not the only factors. In enabling people to access opportunities, we must move beyond 'changing the individual to fit in'. Changing the world so that it can accommodate people with mental health problems is equally important. We must place at least as much emphasis on the provision of support, changing the social and physical environment, changing attitudes, and modifying expectations.

VALUING PEOPLE

If we are to help people to avail themselves of opportunities outside the mental health services, we have to believe in them and in their right to access the facilities and activities that we ourselves enjoy. This can present challenges for our personal, as well as our professional, lives. Bumping into a client in the local pub or church erodes the safe social distance between the 'them' and 'us' attitude to which we have become accustomed. 'Promoting social inclusion' is easy in the abstract, but when faced with its reality in our own neighbourhood it becomes more challenging. Our fine principles may be tested. We may go to great lengths to ensure that supported accommodation can be built in someone else's street, but what if it is next door? People with mental health problems are not dangerous, but what if it is our children that they are talking to in the street? Roles can become confused. What does it do for our 'professional relationship' for a client to see us arguing with our children in the supermarket, or out drinking in the local pub, or at a party with our mates? Challenging myths and misunderstanding is easier in others than in ourselves, but the real challenge to inclusion may be closer to home.

Section 4

Changing the balance of power

12

Involving service-users in mental health services

This book has focused on individuals, on the challenges faced by people with mental health problems in rebuilding their lives, and on the ways in which mental health workers can assist. But recovery does not happen in a vacuum. It occurs in the social context of widespread prejudice and discrimination within mental health services and the wider society. If mental health workers are to facilitate recovery our vision must extend beyond the individual to the services in which we work and the communities in which we live. Far–reaching changes are required if people are to access the opportunities they need to rebuild their lives. These essentially involve changing the balance of power.

In this chapter, we address ways in which the balance of power can, and is, being changed within mental health services. In the next chapter, we move on to consider issues of power in a wider society.

A CHANGE OF FOCUS WITHIN MENTAL HEALTH SERVICES

If services are to promote recovery, the expertise of people who have faced mental health problems must be the primary force guiding their development. Unless the concerns of service-users can be tapped, it is not going to be possible to develop services that enable them to rebuild valued and satisfying lives. This means that a major shift is needed in the values and practices of mental health services and those who work within them. The need for such a change in focus lies at the core of the Department of Health's (2000a) *NHS Plan*, the fundamental aim of which is to reshape services from the perspective of those who are on the receiving end of our ministrations:

> *Patients are the most important people in the health service ... Too many patients feel talked at, rather than listened to. This has to change. NHS care has to be shaped around the convenience and concerns of patients.*

To bring this about, patients must have more say in their own treatment and more influence over the way the NHS works. (Department of Health 2000a)

This is not the first time that the need for such changes has been identified in UK mental health policy. The consumerism which permeated the National Health Service in the 1980s attempted to create actual or quasi 'internal markets' and resulted in increased attention to the voice of the 'consumer'. In 1985, the House of Commons Select Committee on Community Care remarked on 'the difficulty we have had in hearing the authentic voice of the ultimate consumers of community care' and recommended that 'all agencies responsible ensure that plans for services are designed *with* as well as for mentally disabled people and their families' (our emphasis).

Shortly before he became Chief Executive of the National Health Service, Alan Langlands told the Health Select Committee of Inquiry into Mental Health Services that, 'We are listening to carers and users, the people whom we think know best about services.' (House of Commons Health Select Committee 1993). This sentiment was echoed by David King, Chair of the National Health Service Executive's Mental Health Task Force established in the early 1990s:

The work of the Mental Health Task Force has had three strands: to listen to service users, to discover from them what is good and what is not so good about mental health services – what works well for them and what does not; to identify and disseminate examples of good practice services that offer people who use them what they need; and to devise ways of improving performance so that people in every area have access to the best mental health treatment and support. (Mental Health Task Force 1995)

Similar intentions have been reiterated in subsequent policy directives, e.g.:

Patients, service users and carers will be involved in their own care and in planning services. (*Modernising Mental Health Services: Safe, Sound and Supportive,* Department of Health 1998)

Patients provide a uniquely valuable perspective on services, and it is impossible to get the best from the change process without actively involving them. (Department of Health 1999)

People with mental health problems can expect that services will involve service users in planning and delivery of care. (Department of Health 1999)

Although major national user networks such as Survivors Speak Out and the UK Advocacy Network were founded in the mid 1980s, it would be a mistake to assume that 'user involvement' was simply a creation of National Health Service consumerism (Campbell 1996c). The history of protest by people labelled 'insane' stretches back to the second half of the 19th century (Campbell 1996b, c, Sayce 2000) with the Alleged Lunatics Friendly Society. In the 1870s, the work of early feminists such as Georgina Weldon (*How I Escaped the Mad Doctor*) and Rosina Bulwer-Lytton (*The Bastilles of England: Or The Lunacy Laws at Work* – see Showalter 1985) offered critiques of psychiatry as a means of social control. A century later, the user activism that developed in the context of the 1970s Civil Rights Movement (following the lead of black, women's and gay/lesbian groups) is described in Judi Chamberlin's (1977) ground-breaking book *On Our Own*. Although this text was not published in the UK until 1988, the UK Mental Patients' Union was active in the 1970s, and the early 1980s saw the birth of campaigning groups such as the British Networks for Alternatives to Psychiatry and the Campaign Against Psychiatric Oppression.

Within the user movement, two distinct trends can be distinguished (Perkins & Repper 1998): (1) a radical, anti-psychiatry movement concerned with the right to reject psychiatric services and provide user-controlled, user-run alternatives outside the mainstream psychiatric enterprise; and (2) a reformist user/consumer movement whose focus is on improving existing mental health services and campaigning for more involvement and control within them. Perhaps because we, ourselves, are firmly embedded within mainstream services, the primary focus of this book is on these latter endeavours, i.e. ways in which existing statutory and voluntary service-providers can better facilitate the recovery of those whom they serve. However, we would not argue for the primacy of such reforms over more radical endeavours. As long as most people with mental health problems come into contact with mainstream services, work to improve these is important. However, when people become involved in services, they are inevitably influenced by the traditional models and practices that prevail. It is difficult, if not impossible, both to work within existing services and sustain the independent, critical stance that may be necessary to bring about more radical alternatives.

The changed political climate of the 1980s undoubtedly allowed small, independent, user/survivor action groups – especially those with a less confrontational approach – to flourish and grow into thousand-strong national, regional and global networks (Campbell 1996b,c). The efforts of such organisations have undoubtedly resulted in changes:

◆ Service-users have been involved in numerous local planning groups and nationally in the Department of Health's Mental Health Task Force, the National Reference Group which developed the 1999 National Service Framework for Mental Health, and the development of the National Institute for Mental Health England (NIMHE).

◆ Numerous 'patients' councils' and 'user forums' exist within individual services.

◆ Recipients of mental health services are increasingly employed within services as user development workers, consultants and clinicians (Perkins 1998).

◆ In many areas, service-users are involved in staff selection and training (Mental Health Task Force 1994, Sainsbury Centre for Mental Health 1997), research (Rose 1996, Faulkner & Layzell 2000) and service monitoring/evaluation (East Yorkshire Monitoring Team 1997, Rose 2001).

◆ A variety of methods have been developed to facilitate user involvement in individual care planning and delivery (Leader 1995, Avon Measure Working Group 1996; National Schizophrenia Fellowship 2000).

◆ Chamberlin's (1977) call for the creation of user-run alternatives to mainstream services has been realised in numerous initiatives in the USA and, to a lesser extent, the UK (Lindow 1994, Barker & Peck 1996).

Yet, at the start of the 21st century, there remains a great deal of ambivalence towards the involvement of service-users:

On the one hand professional organisations publicly encourage greater involvement of service users (and carers) and acknowledge the legitimacy of direct experience; however, on the other there is a resistance to non-expert views. In the same way that society is uncertain about the new population of patients living in their midst, many mental health workers are wary of those service users now involving themselves in mental health service development. (Campbell 2001b)

It remains rare for people with mental health problems to exert a significant influence over either the development of services or their own care and support within them (Perkins & Goddard 2002). A great deal of 'user involvement' remains essentially tokenistic:

◆ Users may be given copies of their care plans and asked to sign them, but the content remains largely determined by professionals.

◆ Many 'community meetings' and 'user forums' within services do little more than decide on the destination for the next 'outing' or the colour of the walls, or simply offer an opportunity for staff to explain why they cannot respond to service-users' requests. They may also provide a forum where workers can 'provide feedback': too often, this means 'telling people off' for not doing things in the way in which they were supposed to (e.g. they failed to clean the bath, or they played music too loudly).

◆ The one or two 'user representatives' in planning meetings full of senior managers have little option but to accept the agendas and priorities set by service-providers.

As Campbell (1996a) concluded, while the credibility and respectability of people with mental health problems may have increased, there has been little increase in their choice of services or control over treatments received.

If the rhetoric of 'user involvement' is to become a reality then a major culture change is required on the part of mental health workers. A move away from traditional notions of 'professionalism' in which the 'expert professional' determines what is 'best' for his/her 'patients'. The assumption that the 'professional knows best' is based on the belief that the mental health workers have access to a specialist body of knowledge that cannot be understood by non-professionals. Such assumptions are probably the greatest impediment to genuine user involvement. If professionals believe they know best, then 'involving service-users' is reduced to persuading them of this fact. No real involvement or partnership is possible without mutual respect and acknowledgement of the expertise possessed by both parties. This can only become a reality if our view of professionalism changes. It is not the case that professionals lack expertise, rather that they do not have a monopoly on wisdom. The real challenge we face as practitioners involves placing this expertise at the disposal of those with mental health problems rather than making decisions for them.

WHAT SORT OF INVOLVEMENT?

The term 'user involvement' has been used to refer to a broad spectrum of activities (Campbell 2001a):

◆ an activity where service-users really have the power to choose and initiate action
◆ an activity where service-users are involved at the invitation of service providers
◆ an activity where service-users do not really want to be involved but are cajoled or persuaded by mental health practitioners.

In some ways, people who use mental health services have always been 'involved' in the running of them. In the days of the old asylum, inmates polished the ash trays and ran errands for matron, but this is not the kind of involvement that would be considered legitimate today. Essentially, the *NHS Plan* (Department of Health 2000a) requires a move towards a position in which service-users really do have the power to choose what services they want and to initiate action to change services at a number of levels:

◆ At the individual level, there should be involvement in decisions about the treatment and support people need and the ways in which it is provided.
◆ At the operational level, there should be involvement in decisions about the ways in which facilities/teams are run and in monitoring their operation.

There should be feedback about treatment and support received to inform improvements in service quality.

◆ At the strategic level, there should be involvement in decisions about the range of services to be provided and the planning of services as a whole.

◆ At the research level, there should be involvement in defining the desired outcomes of interventions, evaluating effectiveness in terms of these criteria, and devising/testing new approaches.

There is a world of difference between involvement at an operational, strategic or research level and involvement in the planning and delivery of one's own individual care. A person can choose to participate, or not, in the former, but his/her care will be planned and delivered whether or not he/she elects to participate in the process. It is also important to accept that 'non-involvement' is a legitimate choice. Good services are a right and cannot be contingent upon involvement. Mental health workers and managers are responsible for improving the quality of services whether or not those who receive them choose to become directly involved in the improvement process.

Involvement is easy when workers and service-users agree. The real challenge occurs when a service-user wants something that the practitioner considers suboptimal or potentially damaging. It is often argued that services should 'empower' those who receive them, but multiple meanings of the term 'empowerment' can be discerned. Within mental health services 'empowerment' may mean making it possible for people to exercise control over what happens to them, or it may mean a sense of self-esteem with no more actual power (Perkins & Repper 1998). However, it is important to recognise, and be honest about, the very real power differentials that exist.

> *The psychiatric system is founded on inequality. By and large the user is at the bottom of the pile. Our unequal position is symbolised by the compulsory element in psychiatric care. I do not intend to argue for or against the use of legal compulsion in treatment. But the fact of its existence has repercussions for all service users ... That an individual can be compelled to receive psychiatric treatment affects each inpatient regardless of whether their stay is formal or informal ... the threat of legal compulsion nay be used to coerce individuals to accept particular treatments.* (Campbell 1996a)

Policy directives in the mental health arena are replete with conflicting agendas. On the one hand, mental health workers are supposed to provide services that accord with users' wishes and preferences. On the other hand, we are required to minimise risk and protect the public. The existence of mental health legislation – with its provisions for compulsory treatment and detention – sets formal limits on people's rights to make decisions for themselves.

The literature on involvement encourages partnerships between those who provide services and those who receive them. But 'partnership' implies an equality and mutuality that does not exist in mental health services. It is typically providers who invite service-users into partnerships, not the other way around, and their opinions are only heeded in so far as providers wish.

The possibility of compulsory treatment enshrines power differentials and prevents real partnership, but this does not completely eliminate the possibility of mental health workers acceding to service-users' wishes. Nor does it prevent other valuable, and valuing, forms of relationship. Hope-inspiring relationships between practitioners and people with mental health problems require a change in traditional beliefs and practices. It is possible for us, as practitioners, to break down the barriers between 'them' and 'us'. We can listen to the views of those who use services – including people who are compulsorily detained – and change our practices on the basis of what we hear. In order to do this, however, there are certain things we need to do:

◆ We need to recognise user expertise and positively draw on it.

◆ We need to be honest about what is possible and what is not. Everyone's choices are constrained, but if choice is to be meaningful then it is important that these constraints are clear.

◆ We need to ask to what extent the values that inhabit mental health services reflect those of the people who use them.

Our values as mental health workers are at least as important in determining the extent to which people can influence what happens as the structures within which we operate. The critical issue is whether or not we value what service-users have to say, especially when these views differ from our own ideas about what is best:

> *What is important is not so much the mechanisms you erect, but the banners they are assembled under. We all know that involvement in the name of collaboration and in the name of compliance are different things. Involvement can be good or bad, creative or conservative. It is the values motivating the process that are important.* (Campbell 2001a)

PROMOTING MEANINGFUL INVOLVEMENT IN INDIVIDUAL CARE PLANNING

If service-users are to be involved in planning their own treatment and support, then the first requirement is information. Yet the chorus of complaints about lack of information continues unabated:

Most basically, if it is not known that something is available, it cannot be used, it cannot be chosen. Good information makes effective choice possible . . . . We consistently find information provision falling short of what at least half of users would like and this has to be the benchmark – if users do not feel well informed they will be unable to exercise choice and they will be unable to become involved in their care. (Rose 2001)

Campbell & Lindow (1997) emphasise that full information is essential for the development of empowering relationships between practitioners and service-users. Information should be available in accessible forms and involve a continuous process of giving, discussion and checks to see if it has been understood. On the basis of extensive user-focused monitoring of mental health services throughout the UK, Rose (2001) makes the following recommendations:

♦ All prescriptions for psychotropic medication, including prescriptions from hospital pharmacies, should provide full information on the benefits and side-effects of the drugs.

♦ In-patient units should hold this information in accessible leaflet form for all medications used on the ward.

♦ Non-medical staff who take on a care-co-ordinating role, such as social workers and occupational therapists, should be trained in the main side-effects of common psychiatric drugs.

♦ Community mental health teams should develop central, indexed stores of information concerning community resources, housing, benefits, work projects and advocacy. All staff should have basic knowledge of what these stores contain.

♦ In-patient units should have freely available leaflets on the main resources in their locality.

♦ All information should be provided in the locally spoken languages and in forms accessible to those with sensory impairments.

A person should have time to digest information provided and discuss the implications of different options. While there may be occasions when someone is too distressed to take in all the information he/she may need, it is possible to help him/her to consider the different options available when the distress has diminished. It is also possible to help people think, in advance, about the treatment and support they would like when they are in crisis: this takes the form of 'advance directives' or 'advance agreements' (see Chapter 9). A variety of organisations produce information leaflets about the treatment and support options available. [See for example Mind (www.mind.org.uk), the Manic Depression Fellowship (www.mdf.org.uk), the Mental Health Foundation (www.mentalhealth.org.uk), the Depression Alliance (www.depressionalliance.org.uk), the National Schizophrenia Fellowship, now called Rethink (www.rethink.org), and the Royal College of Psychiatrists (www.rcpsych.ac.uk)] Access to written information is important, but it is no substitute for conversation – the opportunity to talk through the pros and cons of different courses of action with a mental health worker, friend, relative or someone else who has similar difficulties.

There are a number of publications that can be used to assist people to become involved in the process of care planning:

◆ *Direct Power* (Leader 1995) was developed by service-users as a resource pack designed to help people to develop their own care plans and support networks.

◆ *The Avon Mental Health Measure* (Avon Measure Working Group 1996) was developed to help service-users to assess their own strengths, wants and needs, express their views to mental health workers, and have more control over the help they receive.

◆ *The Carer and User Expectation of Services questionnaires* (Lelliott et al 1999, 2001, National Schizophrenia Fellowship 2000) were developed as part of the Department of Health's Outcomes of Social Care for Adults initiative. This comprises two instruments – one for service-users, the other for carers – to enable both to contribute to care plans.

Even if they have all the information they need, there are a number of reasons why people may still be reluctant to participate in the care-planning process:

◆ People are unlikely to wish to be involved if they believe their views will not be taken seriously or acted upon. Too often, the process of involvement is experienced as one of being 'talked at' rather than 'listened to'.

◆ Many people are reluctant to criticise the treatment and support offered: 'They may fear repercussions such as loss of service ... that they will be branded as a troublemaker.' (Rose 2001).

◆ If someone cannot see anything of benefit to him/her in the treatment/support options available, he/she is unlikely to wish to become involved in planning the help that is to be received.

◆ The mechanisms used to involve service-users may be difficult to negotiate.

Involving service-users means learning to accept criticism, including criticism that we believe to be unjustified. We must guard against defensiveness and be prepared to reflect on how our often well-intentioned actions may be experienced by those on the receiving end. We need to apologise when we have, albeit unwittingly, caused offence or distress, and change what we do in the light of the feedback we have received. It is *not* a requirement of professionalism that we never make mistakes, simply that we are able to *learn* from them. If we are not prepared to modify what we do, involvement is meaningless.

The mechanisms of care planning also require attention as they can be difficult and unpleasant for the people involved. 'Ward rounds' or 'case conferences' can be extremely daunting. Few of us would want to talk about personal matters in front of a large group of people, some of whom we know only vaguely. Yet this is what such events demand of people with mental health problems. The process could be made less overwhelming in a number of ways:

◆ Meetings can be made smaller by involving only those people directly involved in providing support for the person.

◆ Meetings can be held in a location that is familiar to the person.

◆ The setting can be made more relaxed by, for example, providing comfortable chairs and refreshments.

◆ Notice of who will be attending the meeting and what will be discussed should be given.

◆ The person should be helped to work out what he/she wants to say in advance, and perhaps writing it down if he/she is nervous about speaking in a group setting.

◆ There should be an opportunity for the person to talk privately with key individuals about issues that might be difficult to address in a larger group.

◆ Simple courtesies such as introducing everyone present and making sure that meetings start on time are desirable. Hanging around waiting only serves to increase the person's anxiety.

◆ Language free of jargon and acronyms should be used so that everyone understands what is said. Even commonly used terms, such as 'CPA', mean nothing to the uninitiated.

◆ It should be made clear that the person is welcome to bring along a friend or advocate to help him/her express his/her wishes and concerns.

Many people find it difficult to talk to mental health workers. As Read & Reynolds (1996) said, 'Professionals might not feel very intimidating but there's something about the relationship we have with you. It's not easy for us to say what we want . . . especially when we fear that what we want to say is not what you want to hear.' The assistance of a friend or advocate can help people to say the things they want to say. The *Mental Health National Service Framework* (Department of Health 1999) requires that people have access to advocacy services. Four types of advocacy have been described (Bingley 1990, Perkins & Repper 1998):

◆ 'Self advocacy' is when people represent their own interests and concerns.

◆ 'Peer advocacy' is when someone who has experienced similar problems assists the person to represent his/her views.

◆ 'Citizen advocacy' is when a lay person outside the mental health system represents a person's interests as if they were his/her own.

◆ 'Professional advocacy' is when lawyers or other trained professionals assist people in defending their rights.

In involving service-users in decisions about their own care, the aim must be to enable them to speak for themselves. However, even if someone is able to do this, they may value the opportunity to think through what they wish to say beforehand with a friend or 'advocate'. It may be helpful for the person to write down the things he/she wants to say and the questions he/she wants to ask. Many of us find this helpful in a variety of situations, e.g. when attending a job interview, consulting a lawyer, or going for a hospital appointment.

There are times when most of us seek the support of someone else to help us get our point of view across. Many people have friends or relatives who can help them in this way, but others do not. There may also be times when our wishes conflict with those of the people who are close to us. In such circumstances, an independent 'advocate' can be of assistance. Often people feel more comfortable with someone who has been in a similar situation himself/herself, i.e. a 'peer advocate'. But it is probably the qualities of the 'advocate' that are most crucial, i.e. his/her willingness to understand and effectively represent our views rather than imposing his/her own agenda. There are also times when the advocacy we need requires the specialist expertise of, for example, a lawyer, or welfare-benefits expert. If advocacy is to be effective, it must be independent of the organisation to which the person wishes to express his/her views or concerns. None of us would agree to be represented by a lawyer who was also representing the opposing party. Mental health workers may be able to act as 'advocates' outside the mental health services, helping people to express their concerns to employers or colleges, for example. However, we cannot act as 'advocates' within those services of which we are a part.

Mental health workers may be wary of 'advocates'. We may feel criticised or undermined by them. We may believe that we know the person best and are therefore in a better position to represent their interests, but advocacy can improve relationships between those who provide, and those who receive, services (Leader & Crosby 1998). Given the power differentials that prevail, we must recognise just how difficult it can be for people to express concerns about, or disagree with, someone on whom they rely for support. If we are to improve what we do, those who receive our services must feel confident enough to tell us what is helpful and what is not. Effective advocacy can help people to do this and thereby enable us to improve the treatment and support we offer.

Finally, care plans must be written in a language that is understood by, and acceptable to, the people to whom they relate. A cursory glance through care plans all too often reveals that they are written in a pejorative way using the coded language of psychiatry. For example, one young man came to us in a very distressed state. He said he was not a pervert and that we had no right to accuse him of being one. He showed us a target on his care plan which said 'minimise sexual exploitation'. He believed the term 'exploitation' to be synonymous with 'paedophilia'. When we explained that it meant he should have sex when he wanted to and not when he did not want to, he was much relieved. Had the care plan been written with him, rather than for him, such a misunderstanding could have been avoided.

There may be times when a care plan contains elements with which the person does not agree – as in areas reflecting the requirements of mental health legislation. It is important that the limitations on choice are made clear, but such constraints do not preclude choice completely:

◆ Even where it is necessary to 'agree to disagree', it is important that mental health workers do not simply dismiss the person's dissent. Instead, we should acknowledge it as an understandable response to the person's situation, and formally record his/her perspective.

◆ While a person may not agree with the restrictions imposed upon him/her, there is usually room for negotiation within these boundaries. For example, the nature and timing of medication or leave can be discussed, as can the support and help available while the person is detained.

◆ The care plan should always contain some things that the person wants. It may be possible to help him/her with benefits, provide an opportunity to work out in the gym, or simply bring him/her a cup of tea in bed in the morning. Unless people can see that they are getting something that they value out of the mental health services, there is no reason why they should become involved in them.

INVOLVING PEOPLE IN DECISIONS ABOUT THE OPERATION OF SERVICES

Many things that determine people's experience of using mental health services are determined at the level of the team, ward or unit. The staff team can go a long way to ensuring that people are treated with dignity and respect, that the service is welcoming, and that simple amenities, such as toilet paper, are available. Typically, services look very different depending on whether you are on the providing or the receiving end. The *NHS Plan* (Department of Health 2000a) requires that we improve 'the quality of the patient experience'; if we are to do this, we must understand what services are like from the perspective of those who receive them.

However, it is often the case that mechanisms for involving service-users in individual teams are less well developed than those at a service-wide planning level. In many teams, non-clinical meetings between service-users and staff are a rarity. Onyett et al (1994) found that only 8% of community mental health teams involved service-users in decisions about their teams. Although it is obvious to the team members what the 'multi-disciplinary team' comprises, how it operates, and the range of opportunities that it provides, many of the service-users have only a hazy idea of these things (Meddings & Perkins 1995).

If people are to have a say in the operation of the teams providing their treatment and support, teams need to do the following things:

◆ They need to recognise the importance of such involvement in improving the service provided.

◆ They need to be clear about what they wish to gain from involvement and how they will use the feedback they receive.

◆ They need to furnish the information about the team and its operation that is necessary for involvement. It is particularly important to make clear what can, and cannot, be determined locally.

◆ They need to establish mechanisms via which people can provide feedback on the services they receive.

Feedback may be sought in a number of ways: meetings; open evenings; discharge questionnaires; comments/suggestions boxes; the distribution of postcards that can be returned anonymously asking 'If you could change two things about the service they would be . . .'; and/or the inclusion of people using services at team business meetings. Different people prefer to provide feedback in different ways. Therefore it is often best to use a range of different approaches, but it is important that all are 'user-friendly' and easy to use:

◆ The provision of refreshments, transport and payment can greatly increase the likelihood of attendance at meetings.

◆ The use of external facilitators may increase people's confidence in saying what they really think, as can the opportunity to respond anonymously or speak to someone – independent of the unit/team – whom they trust (e.g. another service-user; see Faulkner & Layzell 2000, Rose 2001).

◆ Stamped addressed envelopes are more likely to be returned than ones which require the sender to pay postage.

◆ Long, complex questionnaires are less likely to be completed than brief, simple ones.

◆ The availability of different languages and formats, and meetings for specific groups who may find it difficult to express their views (e.g. women, people from ethnic minorities), can increase the range of opinions tapped.

Those who will be receiving services should always be involved in project teams charged with the task of developing new services. It is often at this stage that they can have most influence in shaping the service. Such involvement is often best achieved by separate 'user panels' or 'focus groups', which allow the voices of those using services to avoid being eclipsed by professional agendas.

Few people continue to express their views if these are not heeded. It is important that people can see the results of their involvement in the form of at least some changes in practice. In the face of limited resources, a degree of creativity may be required if this is to be achieved. For example, the users of one team asked for access to 'complementary therapies'. Although resources could not be found to employ specialist therapists, it was possible to devote some of the training budget to teaching existing staff members basic aromatherapy and massage skills.

INVOLVEMENT IN SERVICE PLANNING AND DEVELOPMENT

It is now common for one or two service-users to be included in service-wide planning groups such as Clinical Governance committees and National Service Framework Local Implementation Teams. While this may be seen as a positive development, it is often fraught with problems. Service-user representatives:

◆ are often selected on a rather haphazard basis ('I know someone who would be good...') and have no links with local user/survivor groups

◆ often have no means of tapping the views of the constituencies that they are supposed to represent

◆ may be reticent about contributing because they have little or no experience of committee work at this level and find the whole situation rather daunting and overwhelming (something they share with many more junior practitioners in the organisation)

◆ are heavily outnumbered by senior professionals and managers who are extremely experienced in getting their voices heard

◆ have little idea of the remit of the group and its sphere of influence

◆ have little understanding of where the particular group fits in to the overall system and organisational structure

◆ have no way of influencing the agendas of meetings, and are therefore only able to raise issues of concern to them in the last few minutes under 'any other business'

◆ may be told that what they want to discuss lies 'outside the remit' of the group

◆ may find their contributions ignored because it is asserted that they lack the necessary information or 'do not really understand the issues involved'

All of the above means that the ability of service-user representatives to influence what happens is severely constrained.

An increasing number of publications are available which describe how service-providers might effectively involve service-users in planning groups and committees (for example, Voice Your Views 2000, Perkins & Goddard 2002). Campbell & Lindow's (1997) publication *Changing Practice. Mental Health Nursing and User Empowerment* offers advice on involving service-users in the planning of services that is as relevant to other mental health workers as it is to nurses. They emphasise the importance of the process of honesty, clarity, a step-by-step approach and the celebration of success, and offer a comprehensive 'meetings checklist' of things that mental health workers and managers should do if they are inviting service-users to meetings (see below).

◆ *Membership* Service-user representatives should be service-users or ex-users, rather than carers or people from voluntary-sector organisations speaking on their behalf (although these groups may be represented separately, if appropriate, to speak about their own needs).

◆ *Support*
– Service-users should be paid for attending meetings: staff are paid to be there, and service-users should be similarly recompensed for contributing their time and expertise (see McHarron & Nettle 1999, Ryan & Bamber 2002, Scott & Seebohm 2002a,b).
– Travel costs should be paid on the day of the meeting. Many service-users are living on small incomes and can ill afford to wait for the payment of expenses they incur.
– Service-users should have the resources they need to consult other service-users and feed back to them issues raised at the meeting.
– Papers, including the next agenda, should be produced soon after the meeting (rather than immediately before the next one) so that representatives can consult other users.
– Unnecessary paperwork should be avoided.

◆ *Power and decision-making*
– The purpose and limits of the committee should be made clear.
– It should be made clear where the power to make decisions lies.
– It should not be assumed that there are areas in which service-users are not competent to take part.
– Don't pass the buck of difficult or controversial decisions to service-users.
– Service-users should be invited to put items of concern to them on the agenda; such items should not be placed at the end in case there is insufficient time to address them properly.

◆ *At the meeting*
– Jargon should be avoided: practitioners and managers who are present should take responsibility for challenging the use of jargon, as well as being open to challenges from the service-users present.
– Statements should be made about the equality of everyone's contribution at the meeting.
– Issues of confidentiality should be clear.
– It should be clear to practitioners, managers and service-users that no one will be victimised for taking part in consultation and representation. Fear of possible consequences can sometimes prevent service-users saying what they wish to say.
– Drinks should be provided, as many psychotropic medications dry the mouth.
– Practitioners should be prepared for the fact that meetings may sometimes take longer than usual.
– Practitioners should be prepared for strong emotional expression – even anger – and should not regard such expressions as symptoms.
– Regular breaks should be provided for people to have a cigarette, etc.
– Individuals and groups should be told that their input is appreciated.
◆ *Access*
– Meetings should be held in 'user-friendly' and public-transport-accessible places (or transport provided) and at times that are convenient to those involved: people should be asked about these things.
– It should be remembered that mental health service-users may also have physical impairments; meetings should be accessible in this sense as well.

Service-users on committees need to have access to a constituency of the people they are supposed to represent, and to be considered appropriate representatives by these constituencies. It is therefore important to support – both financially and administratively – existing user forums/groups (or new ones if none exist locally) from which representatives can be drawn. Particular attention should be paid to ensuring representation from groups of people who may have specific issues to raise (e.g. older people, younger people, people from ethnic minorities, women, lesbians, and gay men). However, it is also important for mental health workers to offer to attend user meetings, rather than always expecting service-users to come to practitioner-organised meetings.

In order to maximise their influence, mental health professionals and managers adopt a number of strategies. These may be equally important to service-user representatives if their contribution is to be optimised:

◆ *Understanding the prevailing politics* In any situation there are key players who have their own interests and agendas. There are also local and national policy directives to be considered. An understanding of both of these can be useful in deciding where 'windows of opportunity' might lie. The divergent interests of different local stakeholders may offer opportunities for powerful alliances on specific issues.

◆ *Being opportunistic* Most stakeholders, including service-users, have a number of different issues they wish to raise. The key to success often lies in pursuing each at the most opportune time. National and local political imperatives, and the areas in which resources are likely to be available, are important considerations in making such decisions.

◆ *Understanding the decision-making process* Preparatory work outwith meetings can be important. In order for a new idea to be accepted it is often useful to canvas opinion among key people who will be involved in the decision-making process. We, ourselves, have a rule that we do not raise any new issues for the first time in meetings, but instead sound out the views of key participants with the odd telephone call or a chat beforehand. People do not generally like surprises, so gaining information about people's views can help refine answers to any objections that may be raised.

◆ *Accepting that changes may be slow* Revolutions are unlikely to happen in the National Health Service. It is often necessary to 'start small' and gradually chip away at entrenched attitudes and practices.

◆ *Individual examples can be easily dismissed* Personal stories are important in enabling practitioners to understand the experience of using mental health services, but there are limitations to this approach. There is sometimes a rather voyeuristic quality in the response of professionals listening to such stories – a kind of modern-day equivalent of viewing the 'lunatics' at the old 'mad houses'. Precisely because they are individual cases, they are too easily dismissed as being isolated and unrepresentative, for example as a relic of the past 'that doesn't happen any more' or in comparison to someone else: '*I* don't do things like that!'. Often a 'percentages and vignettes' approach can be more persuasive, i.e. supplementing individual, emotive accounts with figures that indicate how many people have had similar experiences. For example, we recently attended a meeting at which a service-user told how, when she was an in-patient, her purse, containing the last remaining picture of her much-loved grandmother, as well as money, had been stolen because staff were unable to find a key for her locker. She then proceeded to describe a survey that her user group had conducted which revealed that some 30% of lockers were without keys. Her personal story served to illustrate the consequences of not having a safe space to keep possessions, but could have been dismissed as a 'one-off' unfortunate instance had she not also presented figures to illustrate the generality of the problem.

RESEARCH, MONITORING AND EVALUATION

Historically, people with mental health problems have been involved in research only as subjects in a process designed and controlled by mental health and research workers. Involvement, in both service monitoring and research, has meant little more than completion of questionnaires or interviews in which professionals have decided what is important, determined the content of the questions, analysed the results, and drawn their own conclusions (Perkins & Repper 1998, Perkins 2001b, Rose 2001). Even the very many patient- and relative-satisfaction scales available have been devised by clinicians and therefore reflect their concerns rather than those of service-users (Ruggeri 1994). However, in recent years this has been changing. An increasing number of methods and instruments have been developed by service-users and used by them in monitoring and evaluating services.

Many practitioners express the intention of empowering service-users, but, as we have already seen, empowerment means different things to different people. Rogers et al (1997) devised a scale to measure empowerment as defined by service-users themselves. A user-researcher began by bringing together a diverse group of service-users who developed a definition of the attributes of empowerment from a user perspective. The user-researcher then constructed and evaluated a questionnaire based on these definitions. Good psychometric properties were demonstrated (internal consistency, construct validity, known group validity). A factor analysis revealed five factors: self-esteem and self-efficacy; power and powerlessness; community activism and autonomy; optimism and control over the future; and righteous anger. The resulting instrument therefore offers a way of evaluating the extent to which services are successful in achieving the user-defined goal of empowerment.

However, the expertise of personal experience does not have to be restricted to the determination of outcome measures. The person asking the questions can significantly influence the responses obtained: Service-users often express understandable concerns that the services they receive may be adversely influenced by the answers they give. In assessments of user preference and satisfaction, people often endeavour to please the questioner by saying what they wish him/her to hear (Srebnick et al 1990, Rose 2001). This can be avoided by involving service-users as researchers. People who have themselves experienced mental health problems, who are trained to perform assessments and interviews, are more likely to inspire the trust and confidence of other service-users and obtain richer, more accurate information about their concerns.

Such an approach has been used to good effect in the UK by, for example, user-researchers at the Mental Health Foundation (Faulkner Layzell 2000) and the Sainsbury Centre for Mental Health (Rose 2001). These approaches are user led at all stages from the definition of issues and methods of investigation, to the analysis and reporting of results. It is important to remember that people who use services have many skills. There is an increasing number of people who have both research qualifications and mental health problems who are able to provide the combination of technical skills and personal experience necessary to conduct good user-focused research.

Rose (2001) and her colleagues have developed 'user-focused monitoring'. This is a systematic approach which provides both quantitative and descriptive information about what service-users think about hospital and community services. This approach:

> ...has service users at its core...It empowers users by giving them real work as interviewers. It enabled the voices of the most disabled users to be both heard and have an influence on care delivery....it provides more accurate sensitive information about users' experiences of mental health services than do traditional, professional approaches. (Rose 2001)

It is 'user-focused' in at least five ways:

◆ The research and evaluation is centrally co-ordinated by users and ex-users of psychiatric services who also have professional qualifications.

◆ The instruments are constructed by groups of local service-users who are in touch with 'grass roots' services.

◆ Local service-users are trained to carry out the practical research work, e.g. one-to-one interviews, site visits and focus groups.

◆ 'Informants' are people who make heavy use of psychiatric services, i.e. those people with severe and enduring mental health problems who are often denied a voice.

◆ The results are interpreted and reports written from a service-user perspective (that of the qualified user co-ordinators of the programme).

Although many practitioners may not have access to skilled user-researchers, it is always possible to find out what people with mental health problems want from the treatment and support they receive and to evaluate effectiveness in these terms. Many services have now instituted programmes designed to train service-users to collect data, and it is always possible to ask those people who have experienced mental health problems what they conclude from the results. Real user involvement in monitoring, evaluation and research moving beyond the distribution of professionals' questionnaires to a situation in which service-users direct the whole process.

THE MAGNITUDE OF THE TASK

If mental health services are to respond to the needs and preferences of those who use them, then service-users must be genuinely involved at every level.

'User involvement' cannot be seen as a simple 'add-on' to existing ways of working. As mental health workers, we must recognise the major change in culture and practice that is necessary if the power of service-users to determine the shape and content of services is to increase. This change involves:

◆ a shift from secrecy to openness and sharing of knowledge and information

◆ acceptance of the limitations of our skills and the value of the expertise of personal experience

◆ recognition that some of the things we do, however well-intentioned, may be harmful

◆ willingness to listen and learn from those whom we serve

◆ an ability to reflect on our practice and change what we do.

Perhaps the biggest challenge is to change our understanding of what it means to be a 'professional'. Traditionally, we have used our expertise to make decisions about what is best for 'our clients'. Now the challenge is to put our skills at the disposal of people so that they can make decisions for themselves.

13

Challenging discrimination: promoting rights and citizenship

Though a simple aspiration for most people socially isolated by mental illness, the sense of belonging to a community with all that this can imply for mutuality and participation remains stubbornly elusive in spite of community care. (Morris 2001)

If mental health services are to assist the recovery of the people who use them, then the way in which these services operate is important. Such services, however, and the people who work in them, cannot be separated from the broader social context in which they exist.

The prejudice and discrimination associated with mental health problems have a profoundly negative impact on people with mental health problems, in both direct and indirect ways. First, the social exclusion which results means that people with mental health problems are denied the rights and opportunities that are available to non-disabled citizens. It is very hard to rebuild your life if, everywhere you turn, you face barriers that make it difficult for you to do the things you want to do (see Chapters 2 and 3). Second, prejudice and discrimination limit the scope for changing mental health services. Mental health workers cannot help but be influenced by the prevailing views of the society in which we live, and the prejudice and discrimination of the electorate heavily influence governmental mental health policy. The *Mental Health National Service Framework* (Department of Health 1999) and the *NHS Plan* (Department of Health 2000a) tell us that we must organise services around the needs and wishes of those who use them. At the same time, however, we are required to protect those people whom, it is often assumed, cannot make decisions for themselves, and to protect society from the dangers it is assumed they present (see Perkins 2001c).

There is, however, increased recognition, among both people who experience mental health problems and mental health workers, of the need to address the negative stereotypes that underpin discrimination and exclusion. As user/survivor consultant and activist Peter Campbell (2000) wrote:

> *The great irony of service user action in the past 15 years is that while the position of service users within services has undoubtedly improved, the position of service users in society has deteriorated. As a result, it is at least arguable that the focus of user involvement needs adjustment.*

These sentiments were echoed by Professor Norman Sartorious at the first World Psychiatric Association Conference on Stigma and Discrimination: 'There is no greater problem in the field of mental health internationally than stigma. (Sartorius 2001).

Acknowledgement of the devastating impact of prejudice and discrimination within our society has led to a growth in the number of campaigns designed to combat the negative images of people with mental health problems. Many mental health workers have inevitably become involved in challenging 'nimby' ('not in my back yard') campaigns organised by people who do not want mental health facilities located in their area (Repper et al 1997). A number of local initiatives have sought to promote more positive views of people with mental health problems, and national campaigns have been organised. In 2001, the Department of Health launched the 'Mind Out for Mental Health' campaign which focused on decreasing stigma and discrimination in the workplace and among young people. Similar initiatives have been launched by professional groups such as the Royal College of Psychiatrists, who created the 'Every Family in the Land' programme. In September 2001, the World Psychiatric Association organised the first major international conference on the issue – 'Together Against Stigma' – which brought together many such programmes from around the world.

THE NATURE OF STIGMA

Most definitions of stigma focus on some characteristic of an individual that is devalued. For example, Goffman (1963) defined stigma as 'an attribute that is deeply discrediting' while Cocker et al (1998) described how 'stigmatised individuals possess, or are believed to possess, some attribute, or characteristic, that conveys a social identity that is devalued in a particular social context'. However, use of the term 'stigma' has attracted much criticism.

Oliver (1990) argued that the concept of stigma focuses attention on the perceptions of the individuals at the expense of an examination of the pervasive and socially constructed exclusion from social and economic life that people experience. As such, stigma is unlikely to be a useful concept on which to base efforts to combat the discrimination and exclusion faced by disabled people, because it is unable to '... throw off the shackles of the individualistic approach to disability with its focus on the discredited and the discreditable.' (Oliver 1990). Sayce (1998, 2000, 2002) and Chamberlin (2001) have extended these arguments more specifically in relation to mental health.

Sayce (1998) argues that the terms we use lead to 'different understandings of where responsibility lies for the 'problem' and as a consequence to different prescriptions for action.' Contrasting the concepts of 'stigma' and 'discrimination', she argues that stigma focuses attention on people who are the recipients of rejection and exclusion rather than on those who perpetrate the unjust treatment. This leads to a focus on the impact of stigma on the individual (they are unable to get a job, study, etc.) rather than the mechanisms that result in these disadvantages. She draws parallels with work to combat racism, which has focused on the individual and institutional perpetrators of racism rather than on the individual's experience of the stigma of being black. As Chamberlin (2001) argues, 'the concept of 'stigma' is itself stigmatising. It implies that there is something wrong with the person, while 'discrimination' puts the onus where it belongs, on groups and individuals that are practising it.'

On the basis of arguments such as these, Sayce (1998) believes that people with mental health problems can learn much from the broader disability movement:

'Stigma' has not provided a rallying point for collective strategies to improve access or challenge prejudice. Instead the disability movement has turned to structural notions of discrimination and oppression... the main issue at stake is that we should root thinking and practice in an analysis of unfair treatment.

In the mental health arena, the approach taken by many 'anti-stigma' campaigns has been to educate various sectors of 'the public', telling them that 'mental illness is an illness like any other' – a 'disease of the brain'. It is assumed that if people with mental health problems are viewed as ill in the same way as someone with asthma or diabetes, then negative stereotypes will be eroded and people will not be blamed for their difficulties. However, does the belief that mental illness is an illness like any other reduce discrimination? An increasing body of evidence suggests that it has the reverse effect (Sayce 2000, Read & Harré 2001). As Nordt et al (2001) concluded on the basis of their research in Switzerland, 'Anti-stigma campaigns that focus on the recognition of illness and its particular symptoms run the risk of increasing discrimination.'

The 'illness like any other' approach fails to recognise the prevailing assumption that people with 'brain disease' are 'unable to think properly', 'irrational', 'out of control'. Therefore they are unable to take responsibility for their actions and are likely to be unpredictable and dangerous. These are precisely the negative stereotypes that underlie the discrimination that people with mental health problems experience. Chamberlin (2001) argues that a fundamental problem with many 'anti-stigma' campaigns lies in the adoption of a 'brain disease' model. The person is seen as being marked by his/her disease. At best, such an approach is likely simply to replace fear and hate with pity. Victimhood provides no basis for growth, recovery and citizenship. As Sayce (2000) put it, 'Disabled people want rights, not pity. The pathetic image of the child on the poster has been thrown out along with the telethons and patronising attitudes: 'Piss on pity', ran one movement headline . . .'

THE AETIOLOGY OF DISCRIMINATION

In response to such criticisms of the term stigma, Link & Phelan (2001) undertook a major reconceptualisation of the term. We would agree with those who criticise use of the term 'stigma', and have chosen to use the terms 'prejudice' and 'discrimination'. These focus attention on people and institutions whose behaviour results in exclusion of people with mental health problems from social and economic life. However, following Sayce (2002), we would argue that Link & Phelan's (2001) reconceptualisation of 'stigma' offers a useful analysis of the processes involved in discrimination and exclusion. In their model, Link & Phelan (2001) describe the convergence of a number of interrelated components.

Distinguishing and labelling human differences

This process necessarily begins with the identification of differences between people: intelligence, height, weight, eye colour, mental health status, and so forth. However, the labelling of difference alone does not result in exclusion and denial of rights. Some differences lack social salience and are largely ignored (e.g. the colour of one's car or the length of one's forearm), many others (e.g. food preferences or hair colour) are relevant in relatively few situations, but some characteristics are highly salient (e.g. sexuality, IQ, skin colour and mental health status).

Stereotyping: linking labelled people to undesirable characteristics

After labelling of the differences comes the linking of negative attributes to these labels. The label 'mental illness' has been associated with a number of undesirable characteristics such as dangerousness, unpredictability and incompetence.

The separating of 'them' from 'us'

Those to whom negatively loaded labels are attached are then separated from the rest of society. They are seen as a distinct class of person. There are 'them' (who have mental health problems) and 'us' (who do not). In the process of separation, the negative attributes ascribed to distinguish 'them' from 'us' are elaborated and extended and 'they' become the thing that they are labelled (Estroff 1989). Instead of 'people with schizophrenia, anorexia, mental health problems' 'they' become 'schizophrenics', 'anorexics', and 'the mentally ill'. It is noteworthy that this process is far more marked for people with mental health difficulties than for those with other illnesses. 'Mental illness' is not seen as 'an illness like any other'. People have cancer, heart disease or influenza, but they remain one of 'us' who happens to be ill. But people are 'psychotics' or 'manic depressives' and are very definitely different from 'us'. These identities eclipse any other attributes that 'they' have. This 'them' and 'us' divide remains alive and well both within mental health services and beyond.

Loss of status, and discrimination

When people are labelled, set apart and linked to undesirable characteristics, a rationale is constructed for devaluing and excluding them. This leads to loss of status and to discrimination. It is this dimension that has been relatively neglected in much of the work on stigma. As Fiske (1998) said, 'documenting discriminatory behaviour has not been their strong suit.' Three types of discrimination can be discerned:

◆ *Individual discrimination* is when, for example, people are turned down for a college course because they have experienced mental health problems, or are avoided in the bus queue because they are behaving in an unusual manner, or are taunted/assaulted because they are known to use mental health services.

◆ *Structural discrimination* (akin to institutional racism) exists in the accumulated set of institutional practices that work to the disadvantage of people with mental health problems. For example, people may experience difficulties in getting a job, and therefore become unemployed for protracted periods of time. Such unemployment means that these individuals lack the good work history, references and personal recommendations that are generally required to get a job. Therefore, their chances of employment are further decreased. Similarly, people's education may be disrupted by their mental health problems. Therefore they lack the qualifications necessary to get jobs, especially the higher status positions with promotion prospects. Unemployment leads to poverty, which results in exclusion from social and cultural activities (which invariably require the person to have money). If people cannot afford to go out with friends, or join a sports club, then their social contacts and activities are curtailed. Poverty may also render people homeless, or force them to live in a high-crime area, so they are more likely to become victims of crime, thus aggravating the problems.

◆ *Discrimination resulting from the stigmatised person's beliefs and behaviours.* In the face of individual and structural discrimination it is hardly surprising that people lose confidence in themselves. If you are rejected for a number of jobs, then you may come to believe that you are incapable of working and give up applying for jobs. If people reject you when they hear of your mental health problems then you may give up trying to make friends.

THE IMPORTANCE OF POWER

Most importantly, discrimination and exclusion are dependent on social, economic and political power (Link & Phelan 2001):

◆ The power to determine those differences which are salient in a particular culture
◆ The power to ensure that the culture recognises the differences that have been identified
◆ The power to separate 'them' from 'us'
◆ The power to deny 'them' jobs, decent housing, an adequate income, access to education, etc.

The media have the power to promote exclusion, with headlines about 'mad axe murderers' that devalue and demonise people with mental health problems. Employers have the power to exclude people from jobs. People who are not defined as 'mentally ill' have the power to get together and organise 'nimby' campaigns.

People defined as 'mentally ill' have little power to determine the values and practices of the communities in which they live. Organisations for people with mental health problems identify differences between 'service-users/survivors' and 'mental health professionals'. They have linked those labelled as 'mental health professionals' with characteristics they consider undesirable, e.g. as agents of social control who deprive people of their liberty and forcibly medicate them with toxic substances. They have separated 'us' (users/survivors) from 'them' (mental health professionals). They have excluded 'them' in so far as they can by rejecting their diagnoses and treatments and campaigning against their right to compulsorily detain and treat 'us'. But people with mental health problems lack social, economic and political power. Therefore such endeavours have had little impact on the prevailing negative stereotypes, nor have they substantially reduced discrimination. Indeed, these very activities have been used as a further rationale for exclusion. The challenge that users/survivors present to accepted psychiatric wisdom is seen as an indication of the 'lack of insight' that accompanies mental health difficulties. Dismissing what people say as a manifestation of their psychopathology is a very powerful way of minimising the impact of any challenge that an oppressed group might make to the way in which its members are defined and treated.

Attempts to decrease discrimination and exclusion cannot avoid issues of power. On the basis of the work of Link & Phelan (2001), and an extensive review of the impact of attempts to reduce discrimination and exclusion, Sayce (2002) argues that initiatives are most likely to succeed if they:

◆ effectively challenge the power that underpins discrimination
◆ aim to transform the beliefs of those who have the power to discriminate, and
◆ work within a comprehensive framework of ongoing anti-discrimination work.

CHALLENGING DISCRIMINATION

Drawing on the wisdom of ancient Greece, Huxley (2001) described two levels at which social inclusion can be considered: 'demos' and 'ethnos'. At the level of 'demos', social inclusion is concerned with rights and citizenship:

> *A nation state can achieve the state of 'Demos' when it is inclusive in its definition and realisation of citizenship and when citizen status leads to equality of social, political and legal rights... Congruence between Demos and any nation state will be highest where social inclusion and social cohesion are maximised, but obviously not when a large proportion of the people of the country are denied full citizenship.* (Huxley 2001)

By contrast, social inclusion at the level of 'ethnos' is concerned not with rights, but with community participation and identification.

> *'Ethnos' refers to a cultural community rather than a national community ... [There are] four components that make up an ethnos community: membership, influence, integration and fulfilment of needs; and a shared emotional connection.* (Huxley 2001)

The elements of ethnos are social-psychological in nature. Communities exist not on the basis of rights but on reciprocal relationships between individuals. Community is therefore a matter of choice, not obligation. It is about identification and social participation – a breaking down of the 'them' and 'us' barriers.

At the level of demos, social exclusion relates to the absence of rights and the presence of discrimination that limits access to employment, housing, health, education, community services and the democratic process. At the level of ethnos, social exclusion is defined in terms of the degree of identification and community participation.

We would argue that, in helping people to rebuild their lives, mental health workers need to address social inclusion at the levels of both ethnos and demos. People need to participate in, and feel part of, the communities in which they live. They also need the rights that ensure they have access to the economic, social and cultural opportunities within those communities. Indeed, we would argue that ethnos and demos are interrelated. People are more likely to be able to be a part of their communities if they have a right to those things that are valued in that community (e.g. decent housing and jobs). However, they are more likely to enjoy these rights if they are seen as a part of those communities and can participate in community opportunities alongside non-disabled citizens.

The majority of this book has addressed social inclusion at the level of ethnos. It has focused on social inclusion at the individual level, exploring ways of enabling people to access the opportunities they seek. We have described some of the ways in which the discrimination exercised by individual employers, colleges, and providers of social and leisure activities might be reduced in order to facilitate access for the individual (Chapters 9 and 10). We have also explored ways in which mental health workers might help foster people's confidence, and help them to challenge the negative stereotypes associated with mental health problems. However, we also need to consider issues of rights and citizenship. Standard 1 of the *Mental Health National Service Framework* (Department of Health 1999) requires that mental health workers contribute to challenging the broader structural discrimination and exclusion that impede recovery. It requires that we 'combat discrimination against individuals and groups with mental health problems and promote their social inclusion.'

Sayce (2002) has described a number of attempts to change the beliefs of those who have the power to discriminate. Some approaches have focused on this labelling component and have attempted to minimise or downplay differences between people labelled 'mad' and those labelled 'sane'. For example, the British Psychological Society (2000) describes mental health as a continuum: 'Mental health and 'mental illness' (and different types of mental illness) shade into each other and are not separate categories.' However, Sayce (2002) identifies three possible reasons for the notable lack of success of this type of approach. First, there is a contradiction between arguing a non-discriminatory position – that having an impairment can be positive – and downplaying that impairment as if it were something to be minimised. Other oppressed groups (women, gay people, black people) have not achieved a reduction in discrimination by minimising those attributes that form the basis of the discrimination they have experienced ('I'm the same as anyone else apart my skin colour, gender, sexual identity'). Indeed, such an approach would be considered positively discriminatory and unacceptable. Instead, they have sought to claim, with pride, their identities as a celebration of devalued identities has been an essential part of their anti-discriminatory positions. Some mental health campaigns have adopted a similar approach, e.g. the Mad Pride movement which describes itself as 'A celebration of mad culture' (Curtis et al 2000). Another initiative organised within some German schools chose not to use messages about illness and instead used more celebratory slogans such as 'Crazy, so what?' and 'Normal to be different.' (Schulze & Richter-Werling 2001).

Second, the general public does not believe the message that there is no real difference between themselves and people with mental health problems (Cumming & Cumming 1957, Jones & Cochrane 1981, Health Education Authority 1997, Rogers & Pilgrim 1997, Sayce 2000). Therefore such an approach is ineffective.

Third, minimising difference may just drive discrimination further 'underground', leaving fundamental beliefs unaltered. Hiding difference carries with it the accompanying risk of being 'found out' when differences are noted.

Other challenges to the beliefs of those who have the power to discriminate have focused on changing the social value attached to particular differences. Indeed, some efforts in this direction have been made in the opening chapter of this book, in which we attempted to replace the ubiquitous stereotypes of incompetence and dangerousness with examples of abilities, creativity and success. However, as Sayce (2002) illustrates, the key lies in the messages with which negative stereotypes are replaced. The lack of success of using an 'illness like any other' message to replace existing negative stereotypes illustrates the importance of properly evaluating the impact of alternative images.

It is also the case that stereotypes are difficult to shift. More positive images frequently have to compete with powerful messages that reinforce existing stereotypes. This is illustrated by the experience of one World Psychiatric Association anti-stigma pilot programme in Calgary, Canada. In this initiative, attempts were made to ensure an increase in the number of positive stories about people with mental health problems appearing in local media. These attempts were successful: the number of positive stories increased by 35%. But at the same time, 'negative stories' of the 'psycho-killer' variety increased by 44% (and included the murder of a police officer, and the American 'Unabomber') (Warner 2000).

One of the most direct ways of challenging the separation of 'us' and 'them' is by achieving direct contact between the two categories, enabling people with and without mental health problems to come together on equal terms. One programme within mental health services achieved this via a range of initiatives designed to increase access to employment within the service for people with mental health problems. These ensured that 27% of recruits had personal experience of mental health problems, and people with and without mental health problems worked together on an equal basis (the same positions, terms and conditions, and responsibilities; see Perkins 1998, Perkins et al 2001b). Attempts have also been made to change attitudes outside the mental health services by publicising (on national radio, and in a London newspaper, e.g. Perkins 2001a) this programme's success in enabling people with mental health problems to work successfully in responsible and senior positions.

It is important to note that the attitudes of those in positions of power were critical to the success of this employment programme in lowering the 'them' and 'us' barriers. Similar programmes that have not enjoyed the active support of the Chief Executive and Chairman have been notably less successful (Perkins et al 2000). Such support from those with power may also contribute to the extension of employment opportunities throughout the National Health Service via national initiatives encouraging the employment of people with mental health problems (see Department of Health 2000a, b, 2001a) and positive ministerial statements:

A key objective of the Government is to enable all disabled people, including those with mental health problems, to make the most of their abilities at work and in the wider society and, as the largest public sector employer in the country, the NHS should also be making a significant contribution to delivering this agenda. The South West London and St. George's Mental Health Trust user employment programme is an excellent example of such initiatives. (Secretary of State for Health in Department of Health 2000c)

However, the impact of such initiatives has been relatively limited. If participating alongside people who do not have mental health problems is to be effective in breaking down the 'them' and 'us' barriers, then it is necessary that people know that those with whom they are working, studying or pursuing social/leisure pursuits have mental health difficulties, and that they allow them to participate on equal terms.

If a person is not known to have mental health problems – to be one of 'them' – then his/her presence will not decrease the discrimination. If his/her presence is only allowed on less favourable terms, then this serves to reinforce the difference ('they' are not able to do what 'we' can do). Given the discrimination and exclusion that exist, many people remain understandably fearful about being open about their mental health difficulties. They know that, if they do so, they risk being sacked, shunned by other people in the pub, denied access to higher level college courses, and so on. Even if they are not excluded completely, participation may be permitted only on very unequal terms. At work, they may be restricted to lower level jobs or denied access to promotion. In other settings, their inclusion may be viewed as a 'good deed' on the part of others, i.e. 'helping the poor unfortunates'.

While there are undoubtedly people who seriously want to change the position of people with mental health problems in society, it seems unlikely that discrimination will be substantially reduced by goodwill alone. Interventions from an 'ethnos' perspective are unlikely to be successful without legislation that renders discrimination illegal: 'Education, Education . . . . Litigation' (Sayce 2001a).

We are not suggesting that legislation alone will reduce discrimination, but we do believe that formal, legal rights at the level of 'demos' are an essential component of promoting inclusion. The challenge to discrimination against women and racial minority groups has occurred at the level of both 'demos' and 'ethnos'. Legislation prohibiting discrimination on the basis of race or gender, and commissions to enforce this legislation (the Equal Opportunities Commission and the Commission for Racial Equality) have gone hand in hand with more educative efforts to change attitudes and behaviour (e.g. anti-discrimination campaigns and awareness training). With the 1995 Disability Discrimination Act and the establishment of a Disability Rights Commission in 2000, the beginnings of legislation debarring discrimination on the basis of mental health problems now exists.

ANTI-DISCRIMINATION LEGISLATION: OPPORTUNITIES OFFERED BY THE DISABILITY-RIGHTS AGENDA

The Disability Discrimination Act (DDA) explicitly includes people with mental health problems alongside those with learning difficulties and longer term physical health problems like cancer and AIDs: 'Disability covers everyone who has a physical, sensory or mental impairment including people with heart disease, diabetes, depression, schizophrenia or dyslexia …' (Disability Rights Commission 2001a). However, if this legislation is to be influential in reducing discrimination against people with mental health problems it is vital that people with such problems, and those who work with them, take advantage of the opportunities that it affords. The Disability Rights Commission (DRC) is committed to creating a society in which all disabled people – including those with mental health problems – can participate as equal citizens. It does this by enforcing the law, informing people of their rights and obligations within it, and promoting change through advice and conciliation. These services can be of great benefit to people with mental health problems. [The DRC Helpline telephone no. is 08457 622633 (Textphone 08457 622644), and the website address is www.drc-gb.org.]

For example, one young man with whom we worked applied for an administrative job with the UK Ministry of Defence. He was successful at interview and was offered the job. But this offer was withdrawn following an occupational health assessment that revealed his history of mental health problems. When this happened, his mental health worker told him about the DRC Helpline. She helped him to call and explain what had happened. A member of the DRC 'Case Work' Team wrote a letter to the relevant department of the Ministry of Defence explaining its obligations under the Disability Discrimination Act: in response, it offered him a settlement of £4000.

He could have refused this and pursued his case for appointment with them under the DDA. However, by this time he had already secured another job and was happy to accept the £4000.

In the first four years of the DDA, 23% of the cases taken under its employment provisions involved people with mental health problems. Here, Sayce (2001b) describes some of the notable successes that have been achieved:

> *One case that was settled before tribunal was that of Mr Watkiss. He was offered the job of company secretary with a major construction company, only to have the offer withdrawn when his diagnosis of schizophrenia came to light. He challenged the company under the Disability Discrimination Act and won: the company admitted unlawful discrimination and paid him substantial compensation.*

> *...a woman who applied for a civilian job in a police force as a finger-printing officer was turned down explicitly on the grounds of her mental health problems. She won her case at tribunal.*

> *In 2001 Ms Melanophy – a successful customer services manager in an educational publishing company – won her employment tribunal case. Her performance and conduct had been temporarily affected by her manic depression. Rather than finding out what the problem was, the employer sacked her for gross misconduct while she was absent from work receiving treatment in a psychiatric hospital. The tribunal found that, under the Disability Discrimination Act 1995, the employer had acted 'hastily and prematurely' and had treated her less favourably because of her disability.*

The DDA makes it illegal to discriminate against someone because of his/her mental health problems, but it also requires that employers, education establishments and the providers of goods and services make 'reasonable adjustments' to accommodate, people with such difficulties. This knowledge can be very important to mental health practitioners who are trying to help people with whom they work to access the opportunities they desire. It is not always necessary to resort to legal action to combat discrimination. Often the very existence of legislation is sufficient. The success of any law – from seatbelt requirements to the prohibition of murder – is judged not by the number of successful prosecutions brought within it, but by the number of people who obey it. The primary aim of law is to prevent undesirable behaviour, not to punish offenders after its occurrence.

When we are assisting people to get jobs or access college courses, we have found it very useful to remind employers and colleges of their obligations under the DDA. This can be useful in negotiating changes or adjustments that the person might need in order to do the job or take the course. We have also found the existence of the DDA helpful in encouraging employers and service-providers to take seriously their obligations to people with mental health problems. For example, one London local authority requested that we run training sessions to help senior managers to fulfil their obligations under the DDA to people with mental health problems. The request may have been prompted by the fact that a neighbouring local authority had been required to pay a large settlement to an employee who had taken out a case against it under the DDA.

Disability discrimination legislation does not apply in relation to employment alone, as illustrated by an example relating to one of the authors of this book:

> *When Rachel Perkins sought enhanced disability insurance cover she was refused on the grounds of a diagnosis of manic depression. This was despite numerous promotions and no significant periods of sickness absence, and the fact that the insurance company's medical opinion was formed without their psychiatrist meeting her or even seeing her medical notes. When challenged under the DDA, the company backtracked on its earlier refusal.* (Sayce 2001b)

Once again, the existence of legislation is likely to have had a broader impact than the individual cases pursued within it. For example, the Manic Depression Fellowship has successfully negotiated travel- and life-insurance policies, at very competitive rates, for members with diagnoses of manic depression. Many people with mental health problems are turned down for such insurance or charged very high premiums. (Further information can be obtained from the Manic Depression Fellowship website at www.mdf.org.uk.)

We have also found that knowledge of the existence of anti-discrimination legislation can increase the confidence of people who experience mental health problems and who have hitherto had to accept passively the discrimination they have experienced without the possibility of redress. For example, one woman was reaching the end of her probationary period with a new company. In a previous job, her employment had been terminated after a probationary period and she was sure that this had happened because her employer knew of her mental health problems. Although her supervisor said that her work was good, she was terrified that the same thing would happen again. When told of the provisions of the DDA, her anxiety decreased greatly and she was able to approach her probationary review with much greater confidence.

It is also worth noting that the scope of the DDA is widening. From September 2002, education establishments (schools, colleges, universities, etc.) will have to make reasonable adjustments to accommodate students with mental health problems, and in 2004, the employment provisions will be extended to include most of those employers who are currently exempt, including fire-fighters, police officers, and businesses employing fewer than 15 people. In addition, the DRC is charged with recommending changes and developments in disability legislation to the Government, so there is scope for people with mental health problems and mental health workers to exercise an influence in this area as well. For example, at present it is difficult for some people who have experienced mental health problems to prove employment discrimination because they do not know why they have been turned down for jobs. If a health check is completed before a job is offered, then it can be difficult to determine whether the person was turned down because he/she did not perform well enough at interview or because of his/her mental health problems. This problem could be reduced if employers were required to separate the selection and occupational health processes. If they were required to make a job offer on the basis of application forms and interview and only afterwards perform any necessary health assessment, then discrimination on the grounds of mental health problems would be easier to demonstrate.

Mental health workers can make use of existing disability legislation, and contribute to the development of the disability rights agenda, in a number of ways (see Sayce 2001a,b):

◆ People with mental health problems should be informed of their rights under the DDA.

◆ People should be informed about the assistance available from the DRC Helpline and 'Case Work' Team, and should be helped to access them.

◆ Employers and employees should be helped to decide what 'reasonable adjustments' might be made to facilitate access.

◆ At a more general level, employers, educators and other providers should be informed about the adjustments they might reasonably make for people with mental health problems.

◆ Advocacy initiatives in relation to employment, education, leisure and other services should be provided and supported.

◆ Mental health workers should enter into debates about developments in disability discrimination law to ensure that it adequately serves people with mental health problems.

If we are to assist people to rebuild their lives we must address issues of discrimination and exclusion. In doing this, we have to broaden our vision, looking beyond individual interventions to minimise mental distress and disability. There are many ways in which we can help people to access opportunities on an individual level, but we also have a broader role to play in breaking down the barriers that prohibit such access, for example by making use of anti-discrimination legislation and endeavouring to change the attitudes of those who have the power to perpetuate exclusion.

For people with physical impairments, a major shift in culture has accompanied increased rights. Recent years have seen the England Football Team Manager forced to resign when he made comments insulting to people with physical impairments and the BBC forced to apologise on prime-time TV when athlete Tanni Grey Thompson was unable to get onto the stage to collect her award. Unfortunately, mental health lags behind. No newspaper editors have been forced to resign over prejudiced and derogatory stories about people with mental health problems. It apparently remains socially acceptable for the Foreign Secretary to use psychiatric diagnosis as a term of abuse when describing Osama Bin Laden as a 'paranoid psychotic'. Perhaps we have a role in objecting to such representations? Perhaps we could campaign for new laws to constrain derogatory representations in television series and inflammatory media coverage? Reducing discrimination involves moving outside traditional 'therapeutic' roles, and using our expertise and influence to help change the world in which we live.

14

Conclusion

In this book, we have presented a model of mental health practice in which the primary focus is recovery: enabling people with mental health problems to maintain or rebuild valuable and satisfying lives within and beyond the limits imposed by their difficulties. Such an approach necessarily involves moving beyond a consideration of symptoms and deficits to an understanding of people in the context of their life as a whole, appreciating their abilities, possibilities and dreams, as well as their roles and relationships. We have moved away from a traditional focus on treatments and cures towards a consideration of social inclusion, enabling people who experience mental health problems to do the things they want to do and live the lives they wish to lead.

Within the model that we have presented, the essence of recovery lies not in the removal of mental health problems but in recovering a meaningful and valued life. Recovery does not require that a person's symptoms disappear – this may or may not be possible or desirable – and social inclusion is not contingent on changing people to render them 'normal'. The primary goal must be a society in which all disabled people – both those with physical impairments and those with mental health problems – can participate fully as equal citizens (Disability Rights Commission 2001a,b). The challenge that we face is to enable people with recurring or ongoing cognitive and emotional difficulties to become valued members of their communities and have access to the same opportunities as non-disabled people.

Many of the critiques of traditional psychiatry have challenged the 'medical model' and called for more alternatives to medication in the form of 'talking' and 'complementary' therapies. While we would not deny the need for people to have access to a range of interventions, we would argue that there is a need to move beyond a 'health' perspective – whether this is conceptualised in biological, social, psychological or spiritual terms. People choose to understand their difficulties in many different ways, but all share the prejudice and negative images associated with mental health problems. It is these, not the symptoms and problems themselves, that have such a devastating impact on people's lives. Images of danger and incompetence underpin discrimination and provide justifications for exclusion. This cannot be understood or challenged from within a 'health' perspective of 'treatment' and 'cure'.

In combating discrimination we have much to learn from others who have faced similar challenges: people from ethnic minorities; lesbians and gay men; and people with physical impairments. The broader disability movement did not reject medicalisation in terms of a more acceptable therapeutic approach. They rejected medicalisation in favour of rights, i.e. rights – to employment, to education, to being educated, to travel, to vote, to stand as a politician, etc. And they have made significant gains. While there are many battles left to fight, we have, for example, politicians with physical impairments (just as we now have black politicians or openly lesbian and gay politicians). But where are the politicians with schizophrenia or manic depression? If they exist, they remain firmly 'closeted' for fear of what disclosure might mean in a society that still considers it acceptable to use words such as 'psychotic', 'loony', 'mad', and 'schizophrenic' as terms of ridicule and abuse.

A choice of effective treatments, offered in a respectful manner, is as important to people with physical impairments as it is to those of us with cognitive and emotional difficulties. However, treatment constitutes only a small part of the assistance that people need in order to rebuild their lives, and does not constitute an organising principle for the provision of such assistance. When we think about people with physical impairments, we think first about access and about rights. When we think about supports and services, we think about them in terms of the ways in which they facilitate access and enable people with physical impairments to do the things they want to do. But still, in the mental health world, we put much of our energy and creativity into debating the treatments and therapies available. When we think about rights, our vision is typically limited to the right to refuse such treatments.

It is our contention that, if people with mental health problems are to make the most of their lives, we need to move away from a narrow 'health' perspective to one which focuses on rights, opportunities and citizenship. Treatments may be a part of this but represent only one component amongst many. As mental health professionals, we need to encompass a far broader vision. We have argued that the organising principle of our endeavours should be one of enabling people to retain and rebuild valued and satisfying lives. This principally involves challenging discrimination and promoting inclusion by facilitating access to those opportunities that are important to the people we serve. Such a change in vision is consistent with the requirements of current mental health legislation (Department of Health 1999, 2001b) but requires a shift of emphasis and approach on the part of practitioners. Health legislation currently requires the bringing together of the historically separate 'health' and 'social' care (Department of Health 1999, 2000c). We are obliged to attend to people's 'social' needs as much as their 'health' needs. The 'recovery and social inclusion' model that we have outlined in the pages of this book offers a guiding principle for integrating these health and social care initiatives towards a common aim, namely enabling people with mental health problems to lead the lives they wish to lead.

This type of perspective requires that mental health workers address issues of discrimination at all levels: individual discrimination, structural discrimination, and the discrimination that results from the impact of these on people's confidence and aspirations. It also requires that we envisage the possibilities of a meaningful life with mental heath problems. Like the great civil-rights leader Martin Luther King, we have a dream. As this is the mental health arena, we perhaps have a *vision* of inclusion (Perkins 2000).

We have a vision that those of us with mental health problems can be known for the contribution that we make to the communities in which we live, rather than being the objects of pity, fear or derision.

This vision does not have to be a delusion. Despite discrimination, there are millions of people with mental health problems who are husbands, mothers, friends or colleagues. We are ordinary people with our own homes who work, raise children, and contribute to our communities in so many ways. We are the real 'silent majority' – silent because we are often too scared to tell people about our mental health problems for fear that we will lose the things we hold dear, and silenced because we do not accord with the popular conception that everyone with mental health problems is either dangerous, incompetent, or both.

We have a vision that it is possible to end the national disgrace demonstrated by 82% unemployment among people who experience mental health problems.

This vision does not have to be a delusion. Work is important for many people, and we know many ways of helping people to achieve this ambition: providing intensive support to enable people to get and keep the jobs they want; ensuring effective social security systems that really enable people to work as much as they can by cushioning them against fluctuations in their ability to do so; compensating employers for periods of sickness absence; or supporting user-run businesses. Enormous resources – in the form of state benefits, legions of professionals, and institutions such as day centres – are currently devoted to supporting inactivity and maintaining exclusion. Would it not be preferable to use at least some of these resources to provide the things that would enable people with mental health problems to work and contribute to their communities?

We have a vision that one day those of us with mental health problems will enjoy all the other rights and opportunities that non-disabled people enjoy –

to do jury service, to study, to raise children, to get insurance – that one day we will see a prime minister who talks openly about his/her experience of schizophrenia or manic depression.

This vision does not have to be a delusion. Many people already do jury service and never mention the treatment they are receiving for mental health problems. The Chicago Mothers' Project (Zeitz 1995), shows us how women with serious mental health problems can successfully raise children if they receive the support and help they need. Although he was forced to keep very quiet about it during his term of office, we know that Prime Minister Winston Churchill had recurrent mental health problems. We know from the work of the Manic Depression Fellowship that companies can be persuaded to provide those of us with mental health problems with travel and life insurance without charging grossly inflated premiums.

We have a vision that one day it will be possible to talk openly about mental health problems to friends, neighbours and colleagues without fear of being devalued and excluded and without attracting those delicate 'changes of subject' that indicate that such issues should be kept firmly behind closed doors.

We have a vision that one day derogatory and pejorative descriptions of people with mental health problems – and the use of 'nutter' and 'schizophrenic' as terms of derision and abuse – will be as unacceptable as derogatory racist language.

We have a vision that people with mental health problems will be able to talk of their experiences, dreams and aspirations without these being ignored and written off as unrealistic, lacking in insight, or the ramblings of a deranged mind.

It is very easy for mental health workers to dismiss as an impossible 'pipe-dream' ambitions such as these, or to despair at the hopelessness of the situation of those whom we serve. We may not be able to change the world, but we can use the power and resources available to us – however limited these might be – in the service of a vision of inclusion. There are many ways in which we can help people to retain or regain self-respect and dignity, and to access the opportunities they desire in order to pursue their ambitions. Without a vision of future possibilities, we have no direction for our work and no yardstick against which we can judge our success. If we cannot entertain the possibility that people with mental health problems can participate fully and equally in our communities, can we really say that we value them? Can we really facilitate their recovery? We must aim higher. We must move beyond the aim of community presence embodied in community care initiatives to community membership and participation – to citizenship and rights.

References

Adams S A, Partree D J 1998 Hope. The critical factor in recovery. Journal of Psychosocial Nursing 36:29–32

Aguilar E J, Haas G, Manzanera F J et al. 1997 Hopelessness and first episode psychosis: a longitudinal study. Acta Psychiatrica Scandinavica 96:25–30

Alexander D 1994 A death–rebirth experience. In: Spaniol L, Koehler M (eds) The Experience of Recovery. Center for Psychiatric Rehabilitation, Boston, p 36–39

Allebeck P 1989 Schizophrenia: a life-shortening disease. Schizophrenia Bulletin 15:81–89

Anonymous 1995 The drug treatment of patients with schizophrenia. Drug and Therapeutics Bulletin 33:81–86

Anonymous 2001 Being positive about schizophrenia. Personal experience of schizophrenia. Journal of Psychiatric and Mental Health Nursing 8:269–280

Anthony W A 1977 Psychological rehabilitation. A concept in need of a method. American Psychologist 32:658–662

Anthony W A 1979 Principles of Psychiatric Rehabilitation. University of Park Press, Baltimore

Anthony W A 1993 Recovery from mental illness: the guiding vision of the mental health system in the 1990s. Innovations and Research 2:17–24

Anthony W A 1994 Characteristics of people with psychiatric disabilities that are predictive of entry into the rehabilitation process and successful employment outcomes. Psychosocial Rehabilitation Journal 17:3–14

Anthony W A, Cohen M R, Cohen B F 1984 Psychiatric rehabilitation. In: Talbott J A (ed) The Chronic Mental Patient: five years later. Grune and Stratton, Orlando, p 213–252

Anthony W A, Cohen M, Farkas M 1990 Psychiatric Rehabilitation. Center for Psychiatric Rehabilitation, Boston

Anthony W A, Rogers E S, Cohen M, Davies R R 1995 Relationships between psychiatric symptomatology, work skills and future vocational performance. Psychiatric Services 46:353–358

Appelo M T, Woonings F M J, Van Nieuwenhuizen C J 1992 Specific skills and social competence in schizophrenia. Acta Psychiatrica Scandanavica 85:419–422

'A psychiatric nurse' 1996 I suffered from depression. In: Read J, Reynolds J (eds) Speaking Our Minds. Macmillan, London, p 35–38

Avon Measure Working Group 1996 The Avon Mental Health Measure. A user-centred approach to assessing need. Mind, Avon

Bachrach L L 1982 Assessment of outcomes in community support systems: results problems and limitations. Hospital and Community Psychiatry 40:234–235

Barker P J 1982 Behaviour Therapy Nursing. Croom Helm, London

Barker P J 1992 Psychiatric nursing. In: Butterworth T, Faugier J (eds) Clinical Supervision and Mentorship in Nursing. Chapman and Hall, London, p 56–72

Barker P J 1999 The Philosophy and Practice of Psychiatric Nursing. Churchill Livingstone, London

Barker I, Peck E 1996 User empowerment – a decade of experience. The Mental Health review, 1(4): 5–13

Barker P J, Davidson B, Campbell P 1999 (eds) From the Ashes of Experience. Whurr Publications, London

Bartley M 1994 Unemployment and ill-health: understanding the relationships. Journal of Epidemiology and Community Health 48:333–337

Bauby J-D 1998 The Diving Bell and the Butterfly. Fourth Estate, London

Beale N, Nethercott S 1985 Job-loss and family morbidity: a study of factory closure. Journal of the Royal College of General Practitioners 35:510–514

Bebbington P, Kuipers L 1994 The predictive utility of expressed emotion in schizophrenia: an aggregate analysis. Psychological Medicine 24:707–718

Beck A T, Brown G, Berchick J et al 1990 Relationship between hopelessness and suicide: a replication with psychiatric outpatients. American Journal of Psychiatry 147:11–23

Becker D R, Drake R E 1993 A Working Life. The Individual Placement and Support Program. Dartmouth Psychiatric Research Center, New Hampshire

Bennett D 1978 Social forms of psychiatric treatment. In: Wing J K (ed) Schizophrenia: toward a new synthesis. Academic Press, London, p 56–72

Berman R 1994 Lithium's other face. In: Spaniol L, Koehler M (eds) The Experience of Recovery. Center for Psychiatric Rehabilitation, Boston, p 40–45

Bingley W 1990 An Introduction to Advocacy. Good Practices in Mental Health Information Pack. Good Practices in Mental Health, London

Birchwood M 1992 Early intervention in schizophrenia: theoretical background and clinical strategies. British Journal of Clinical Psychology 31:257–258

Birchwood M, Tarrier N (eds) 1992 Innovations in the Psychologcal Management of Schizophrenia. John Wiley, Chichester

Birchwood M, Smith J, Macmillan F, McGovern D 1998 Early intervention in psychotic relapse. In: Brooker C, Repper J (eds) Serious Mental Health Problems in the Community: policy, practice and research. Baillière Tindall, London, p 204–237

Bird L 2001 Poverty, social exclusion and mental health: a survey of people's personal experiences. A Life in the Day 5:3

Birley J 1999 The nazi experience – past, present or future? Mental Health Reforms 3:3–5

Blackwell B 1972 The drug defaulter. Clinical Pharmacology and Therapeutics 13:841–848

Bockes Z 1989 'Freedom' means knowing you have the choice. In: The Experiences of Patients and Families: first person accounts. Reprinted from Schizophrenia Bulletin and the New York Times. National Alliance for the Mentally Ill, Arlington, VA

Bond G R 1994 Psychiatric rehabilitation outcome. In: The Publication Committee of the International Association of Psychosocial Rehabilitation Services (ed) An Introduction to Psychiatric Rehabilitation. International Association of Psychosocial Rehabilitation Services, Columbia, MD, p 335–345

Bond G R, Drake R E, Meuser K T, Becker D R 1997 An update on supported employment for people with severe mental illness. Psychiatric Services 48:335–346

Bond G R, Becker D R, Drake R E et al 2001 Implementing supported employment as an evidence based practice. Psychiatric Services 52:313–322

Boston Centre for Psychiatric Rehabilitation 2002 What accommodations work on the job? Available online: http://www.bu.edu/cpr/reasaccom/employ-accom.html

Bova S 1995 How do I cope with having a mental illness? The mellow message! Consumer Advocates for Mental Health January/February:12–14

Boyle M 1993 Schizophrenia: a Scientific Delusion? Routledge, London

Breeze J, Repper J 1999 Struggling for control: the care experience of 'difficult patients' in mental health services. Journal of Advanced Nursing 28:1301–1311

Breier A, Strauss J 1983 Self control in psychiatric disorders. Archives of General Psychiatry 40:1141–1145

Brenner M H 1979 Mortality and the national economy: a review of the experience of England and Wales. Lancet ii:685–699

Brenner S, Bartell R 1983 The psychological impact of unemployment. A structural analysis of cross-sectional data. Journal of Occupational Psychology 56:129–136

Brett-Jones J, Garety P, Hemsley D 1987 Measuring delusional experiences: a method and its application. British Journal of Clinical Psychology 26:257–265

British Psychological Society 2000 Recent Advances in Understanding Mental Illness and Psychotic Experience. British Psychological Society, Leicester

Brooker C, Repper J (eds) 1998 Serious Mental Health Problems in the Community: policy, practice and research. Baillière Tindall, London

Brooker C G D, Falloon I, Butterworth T et al 1994 The outcome of training CPNs to deliver psychosocial intervention. British Journal of Psychiatry 165:122–130

Brooks L 1997 Dark side of the star. The Guardian 27 Aug:2–3

Brown G W, Harris T O 1978 Social Origins of Depression: a study of psychiatric disorder in women. Tavistock Publications, London

Brunner E 1972 Eternal Hope. Greenwood Press, Westport, CT

Burchardt T 2000 Enduring Economic Exclusion: disabled people, income and work. Joseph Rowntree Foundation, York

Byrne C, Woodside H, Landeen J et al 1994 The importance of relationships in fostering hope. Journal of Psychosocial Nursing 32:31–34

Campbell J 1989 (ed) People say I'm crazy! Department of Mental Health, Office of Prevention, San Francisco

Campbell P 1996a Challenging loss of power. In: Read J, Reynolds J (eds) Speaking Our Minds. Open University Press, Milton Keynes, p 56–62

Campbell P 1996b The history of the user movement. In: Heller T, Reynolds J, Gomm R et al (eds) Mental Health Matters. Macmillan, London, p 25–31

Campbell P 1996c User action – the last ten years. The Mental Health Review 1:14–15

Campbell P 2000 The role of users of psychiatric services in service development – influence not power. Psychiatric Bulletin 25:87–88

Campbell P 2001a Involving service users in the rehabilitation process. 'Rehab' Good Practice Network Newsletter 4:3–5

Campbell P 2001b The role of users of psychiatric services in service development – influence not power. Psychiatric Bulletin 25:87–88

Campbell P, Lindow V 1997 Changing practice. Mental health nursing and user empowerment. Mind Publications/Royal College of Nursing, London

Chadwick P K 1997a Recovery from schizophrenia: the problem of poetic patients and scientific clinicians. Clinical Psychology Forum 103:39–43

Chadwick P K 1997b Schizophrenia: The Positive Perspective. In search of dignity for schizophrenic people. Routledge, London

Chadwick P, Birchwood M, Trower P 1996 Cognitive Therapy for Delusions, Voices and Paranoia. John Wiley, Chichester

Chamberlin J 1977 On Our Own, 1988 edn. Mind Publications, London

Chamberlin J 1988 Confessions of a noncompliant patient. Journal of Psychosocial Nursing 36:49–52

Chamberlin J 1993 Psychiatric disabilities and the ADA. An advocate's perspective. In: Gostin L O, Beyer H A (eds) Implementing the Americans with Disabilities Act. Brookes, Baltimore

Chamberlin J 1995 Rehabilitating ourselves: the psychiatric survivor movement. International Journal of Mental Health 24:39–46

Chamberlin J 2001 Equal rights, not public relations. World Psychiatric Association Conference 'Together Against Stigma', Leipzig, September 2001

Claridge G S 1985 Origins of Mental Illness. Blackwell, Oxford

Clarke L 1999 Nursing in search of a science: the rise and rise of the new nurse brutalism. Mental Health Care 2:270–272

Cocker J, Major B, Steele C 1998 Social stigma. In: Gilbert D T, Fiske S T (eds) The Handbook of Social Psychology. McGraw-Hill, Boston

Cohen C, Willis T A 1985 Stress, social support and the buffering hypothesis. Psychological Bulletin 98:310–357

Coleman R 1999 Recovery: An Alien Concept. Handsell Publishing, Gloucester

Coleman R, Smith M 1997a Working With Voices. Handsell Publishing, Gloucester

Coleman R, Smith M 1997b Working With Selfharm. Handsell Publishing, Gloucester

Conrad P 1985 The meaning of medications: another look at compliance. Social Science and Medicine 20:29–37

Coursey R D, Curtis L, Marsh D T et al 2000 Competencies for direct service staff members who work with adults with severe mental illnesses in outpatient public mental health/managed care systems. Psychiatric Rehabilitation Journal 23:370–377

Creer C, Sturt E, Wykes T 1982 The role of relatives. In: Wing J K (ed) Long term community care: experience in a London borough. Psychological Medicine (monograph suppl 2):29–39

Cronin-Stubbs D, Brophy E B 1985 Burnout: can social support save the psychiatric nurse? Journal of Psychosocial Nursing 23:8–13

Crowther R E, Marshall M, Bond G R, Huxley P 2001 Helping people with severe mental illness to obtain work: systematic review. British Medical Journal 322:204–208

Cumming E, Cumming J 1957 Closed Ranks. An experiment in mental health. Harvard University Press, Cambridge, MA

Curtis T, Dellar R, Leslie E, Watson B 2000 Mad Pride. A celebration of mad culture. Spare Change Books, London

Cutting J, Murphy D 1988 Schizophrenic thought disorder: a psychological and organic interpretation. British Journal of Psychiatry 152:310–319

Dahrendorf R 1985 The Modern Social Conflict. Weidenfeld and Nicholson, London

Darton K 1998 Genetics Factsheet. Mind Publications, London

Davidson L, Strauss J S 1992 Sense of self in recovery from severe mental illness. British Journal of Medical Psychology 65:131–145

Davis L M, Drummond M F 1990 The economic burden of schizophrenia. Psychiatric Bulletin 14:522–525

Deegan P 1988 Recovery: the lived experience of rehabilitation. Psychosocial Rehabilitation Journal 11:11–19

Deegan P 1989 A letter to my friend who is giving up. In: Proceedings of the Connecticut Conference on Supported Employment, Connecticut Association of Rehabilitation Facilities, Cromwell, CT, USA. Published by the Center for Community Change Through Housing and Support, Trinity College, Burlington, VT, CI-24

Deegan P 1990 How recovery begins. In: Proceedings of the Eighth Annual Education Conference Alliance for the Mentally Ill of New York State, Binghamton, NY, USA. Published by the Center for Community Change Through Housing and Support, Trinity College, Burlington, VT, CI-25

Deegan P 1992 Recovery, rehabilitation and the conspiracy of hope: a Keynote Address. In: Proceedings of the Western Regional Conference on Housing and Support, Trinity College, Vermont. Published by the Center for Community Change Through Housing and Support, Trinity College, Burlington, VT, CI-28

Deegan P 1993 Recovering our sense of value after being labelled mentally ill. Journal of Psychosocial Nursing and Mental Health Services 31:7–11

Deegan P 1996 Recovery as a journey of the heart. Psychosocial Rehabilitation Journal 19:91–97

Deegan P E 1999 Recovery: an alien concept. In: Proceedings of the Strangefish Conference: 'Recovery: an alien concept', Chamberlin Hotel, Birmingham, UK

Department of Health 1998 Modernising Mental Health Services: safe, sound and supportive. Department of Health, London

Department of Health 1999 National Service Framework for Mental Health. Department of Health, London

Department of Health 2000a The NHS National Plan. Department of Health, London

Department of Health 2000b Looking Beyond Labels. Widening the employment opportunities for disabled people in the new NHS. Department of Health, London

Department of Health 2000c The Government's Response to the Health Select Committee's Report Into Mental Health Services, October 2000, Cm 4888. Department of Health, London

Department of Health 2001a Making it Happen. A guide to mental health promotion. Department of Health, London

Department of Health 2001b The Journey to Recovery. The Government's vision of mental health care. Department of Health, London

Department of Health 2001c The National Service Framework for Mental Health Implementation Guide. Department of Health, London

Department of Work and Pensions 2001 Recruiting Benefits Claimants: quantitative research with employers in ONE pilot areas. Research series paper no. 150. Department of Work and Pensions, London

Diamond R J 1983 Enhancing medication use in schizophrenic patients. Journal of Clinical Psychiatry 44:7–14

Disability Rights Commission 2001a Who We Are and What We Do. Disability Rights Commission, London

Disability Rights Commission 2001b Strategic Plan. Disability Rights Commission, London

Donovan J E, Blake D R 1992 Patient non-compliance: deviance or reasoned decision making? Social Science and Medicine 34:507–513

Drake R E, Cotton P G 1986 Depression, hopelessness and suicide in chronic schizophrenia. British Journal of Psychiatry 148:554–559

Dufault K, Martocchio B 1985 Hope: its spheres and dimensions. Nursing Clinics of North America 20:379–391

Duffy K 1995 Social Exclusion and Human Dignity in Europe. Council of Europe, Strasbourg

Dunn S 1999 Creating Accepting Communities. Report of the Mind Inquiry into Social Exclusion and Mental Health Problems. Mind Publications, London

East Yorkshire Monitoring Team 1997 Monitoring Our Services Ourselves: user-led monitoring of mental health services. Beverley, East Yorkshire Monitoring Team

Eisen S A, Miller D K 1990 The effect of prescribed daily dose frequency on patient medication compliance. Archives of Internal Medicine 150:1881–1884

Ekdawi M, Conning A 1994 Psychiatric Rehabilitation – a practical guide. Chapman and Hall, London

Estroff S E 1989 Self, identity, and subjective experiences of schizophrenia: in search of the subject. Schizophrenia Bulletin 15:189–196

Fadden G, Bebbington P, Kuipers L 1987 The burden of care: the impact of functional psychiatric illness on the patient's family. British Journal of Psychiatry 150:285–292

Falloon I, Boyd J, McGill C 1982 Family management in the prevention of exacerbations of schizophrenia. New England Journal of Medicine 306:437–440

Falloon I, Boyd J, McGill C 1984 Family Care of Schizophrenia. Guildford Press, New York

Farkas M, Gagne C, Anthony W A 1999 Recovery and Rehabilitation: a paradigm for the new millennium. Center for Psychiatric Rehabilitation, Boston

Farran C J, Herth K A, Popovich J M 1995 Hope and Hopelessness: critical clinical constructs. Sage Publications, London

Faulkner A, Layzell S 2000 Strategies for Living. A report of user-led research into people's strategies for living with mental distress. The Mental Health Foundation, London

Fehr B 1996 Friendship Processes. Sage Publications, London

Fiske S T 1998 Stereotyping, prejudice and discrimination. In: Gilbert D T, Fiske S T (eds) The Handbook of Social Psychology. McGraw-Hill, Boston

Fleischtaker W W, Meise U, Gunther V 1994 Compliance with antipsychotic drug treatment: influence of side-effects. Acta Psychiatrica Scandinavica 89 (suppl 382):11–15

Ford R, Beadsmore A, Norton P et al 1994 Developing case management for the long term mentally ill. Psychiatric Bulletin of the Royal College of Psychiatry 17:409–411

Foucault M 1967 Madness and Civilisation. A history of insanity in the Age of Reason. Tavistock Publications, London

Francell E G 2002 Medication: the foundation of recovery. Available online: http://www.psychlaws.org/GeneralResources/PA3.htm

Frank J 1968 The role of hope in psychotherapy. International Journal of Psychiatry 5:383–395

Frank E, Kupfer D J, Siegel L R 1995 Alliance or compliance: a philosophy of outpatient care. Journal of Clinical Psychology 56 (suppl 1):11–17

Frese F J 1997 The mental health consumer's perspective on mandatory treatment. In: Munetz M R (ed) Can Mandatory Treatment be Therapeutic? New directions for mental health services 75. Jossey-Bass, San Francisco, p 33–39

Fromm E 1968 The Revolution of Hope. Harper and Row, New York

Gallagher H G 1999 FDR's Splendid Deception. Vandamere Press, Arlington, VA

Galloway J 1991 The Trick is to Keep Breathing. Minerva, London

Garety P 1992 Assessment of symptoms and behaviour. In: Birchwood M, Tarrier N (eds) Innovations in the Psychological Management of Schizophrenia. John Wiley, Chichester, p 14–27

Garrity T F 1981 Medical compliance and clinician–patient relationship: a review. Social Science and Medicine 15:215–222

Glover H 2001 Holders of hope. In: Proceedings of the Focus on Recovery Conference, University of Central England, Birmingham, UK, p 000–000

Goffman E 1963 Stigma: notes on the management of spoiled identity. Penguin, Harmondsworth

Glozier N 1998 Workplace effects of stigmatization and depression. Journal of Occupational and Environmental Medicine 40(9): 793–800

Gourash N 1978 Help-seeking: a review of the literature. American Journal of Community Psychology 6:499–502

Gournay K 1996 Schizophrenia: a review of the contemporary literature and implications for mental health nursing theory, practice and education. Journal of Mental Health and Psychiatric Nursing 3:7–12

Greenberg J S, Greenley J R, Benedict P 1994 Contributions of persons with serious mental illness to their families. Hospital and Community Psychiatry 45:475–480

Grove B, Freudenberg M, Harding A, O'Flynn D 1997 The Social Firm Handbook. New directions in the employment, rehabilitation and integration of people with mental health problems. Pavilion Publishing, Brighton

Harding C M, Zahniser F H 1994 Empirical correction of seven myths about schizophrenia with implications for treatment. Acta Psychiatrica Scandanavica 90 (suppl 384):140–146

Hardman K 1997 My busy mother. Women and Mental Health Forum 2:8–9

Harris E C, Barraclough B 1998 Excess mortality of mental disorder. British Journal of Psychiatry 173:11–53

Hatfield A B 1987 The expressed emotion theory: why families object. Hospital and Community Psychiatry 38:341

Hatfield A, Lefley H 1993 Surviving Mental Illness. Stress coping and adaptation. Guilford Press, London

Hatfield A B, Spaniol L, Zipple A M 1987 Expressed emotion: a family perspective. Schizophrenia Bulletin 13:221–226

Health Education Authority 1997 Young People's Resources to Combat Stigma Around Mental Health Issues. Qualitative research to evaluate resource material. Health Education Authority, London

Heatherton T F, Kleck R E, Hebl M R, Hull J G 2000 The Social Psychology of Stigma. Guilford Press, London

Hickey S S 1986 Enabling hope. Journal of Cancer Nursing 9:133–137

Hogarty G E, Anderson C M, Reiss D J et al 1991 Family psychoeducational, social skills training and maintenance chemotherapy in the aftercare treatment of schizophrenia II: Two year effects of a controlled study on relapse and adjustment. Archives of General Psychiatry 48:340–347

Holdcraft C, Williamson C 1991 Assessment of hope in psychiatric and chemically dependent patients. Applied Nursing Research 4:129–134

Holmes-Eber P, Riger S 1990 Hospitalisation and the composition of patients; social networks. Schizophrenia Bulletin 16:157

Houghton J F 1982 Maintaining health in a turbulent world. Schizophrenia Bulletin 8:548–552

House of Commons Social Services Committee 1993 Health Select Committee Report of the Inquiry into Mental Illness Services. HMSO, London

Hutchinson M, Nettle M 2001 Deciding about disclosure. A Life in the Day 5:30–32

Huxley P 2001 Rehabilitation – the social care dimension. In: Proceedings of the 'Reinventing Rehabilitation' Health Advisory Service Rehabilitation Good Practice Network Conference, London. HAS Rehab Good Practice Network Newsletter 5:2–3

Jackson H J, Smith N, McGorry P 1990 Relationship between expressed emotion and family burden in psychotic disorders: an exploratory study. Acta Psychiatrica Scandanavica 82:243–249

Jacobson N 1993 Experiencing recovery: a dimensional analysis of recovery narratives. Psychiatric Rehabiliation Journal 24:248–255

Jahoda M, Lazarsfeld P, Zeisl H 1933 Marienthal: the sociography of an unemployed community, 2nd edn. Tavistock Publications, London

Jamison K R 1989 Mood disorder and patterns of creativity in British writers and artists. Psychiatry 32:125–134

Jamison K R 1993 Touched with fire: manic-depressive illness and the artistic temperament. The Free Press, New York

Jamison K R 1995a An Unquiet Mind: a memoir of moods and madness. Alfred A Knopf, New York

Jamison K R 1995b Manic depressive illness and creativity. Scientific American 272:62–67

Jones L, Cochrane R 1981 Stereotypes of mental illness: a test of the labelling hypothesis. International Journal of Social Psychiatry 27:99–107

Kanwal G S 1997 Hope, respect and flexibility in the psychotherapy. Contemporary Psychoanalysis 33:133–150

Karlsson J L 1972 An Icelandic family study of schizophrenia. In: Kaplan A R (ed) Genetic Factors in Schizophrenia. Charles C Thomas, Springfield, IL, p 213–221

Keenan B 1993 An Evil Cradling. Vintage Books, London

Kemp R, Hayward P, Applewhite G et al 1996 Compliance therapy in psychotic patients: randomised controlled trial. British Medical Journal 312:315–319

Kemp R, Hayward P, David A 1997 Compliance Therapy Manual. The Maudsley Hospital, London

Kent S, Yellowlees P 1994 Psychiatric and social reasons for frequent rehospitalisation. Hospital and Community Psychiatry 45:347–350

Kingdon D 1998 Cognitive behaviour therapy for severe mental illness: strategies and techniques. In: Brooker C, Repper J (eds) Serious Mental Health Problems in the Community: policy, practice and research. Baillière Tindall, London

Kingdon D, Turkington D 1994 Cognitive Behavioural Therapy of Schizophrenia. Lawrence Ehrlbaum, London

Kirkpatrick H, Landeen J, Byrne C et al 1995 Hope and schizophrenia: clinicians identify hope-instilling strategies. Journal of Psychosocial Nursing and Mental Health Services 33:15–19

Kirkpatrick H, Landeen J, Woodside H, Byrne C 2001 How people with schizophrenia build their hope. Journal of Psychosocial Nursing 39:46–53

Kitzinger C, Perkins R E 1993 Changing Our Minds. Onlywomen Press/New York University Press, London/New York

Kubler-Ross E 1969 Death and Dying. Macmillan, London

Kuipers L 1993 Family burden in schizophrenia: implications for services. Social Psychiatry and Psychiatric Epidemiology 28:207–210

Kuipers E 2001 Involving service users in the rehabilitation process. In: Proceedings of the Rehabilitation Good Practice network Conference, The Russell Hotel, London. HAS Rehab Good Practice Network Newsletter 4:3–5

Kuipers E, Bebbington P 1988 Expressed emotion research in schizophrenia: theoretical and clinical implications. Psychological Medicine 18:893–909

Kuipers E, Moore E 1995 Expressed emotion and staff–client relationships: implications for community care of the severely mentally ill. International Journal of Mental Health 24:13–26

Kumar S, Thara R, Rajkumar S 1989 Coping with symptoms of relapse in schizophrenia. European Archives of Psychiatric Neurological Science 239:213–215

Laing R D 1960 The Divided Self: a study of sanity and madness. Tavistock Publications, London

Landeen J, Pawlick J, Woodside H et al 2000 Hope, quality of life and symptom severity in individuals with schizophrenia. Psychiatric Rehabilitation Journal 23:3464–3469

Lawrence P N 1998 Impressive Depressives. 75 Historical cases of manic depression from seven centuries. The Manic Depression Fellowship, London

Leader A 1995 Direct Power. Pavilion Publishing, Brighton

Leader A, Crosby K 1998 Power Tools. A resource pack for those committed to the development of mental health advocacy into the millennium. Pavilion Publishing, Brighton

Leete E 1988a The role of the consumer movement and people with mental Illness (unpublished). Presentation at the 12th Mary Switzer Memorial Seminar in rehabilitation, June 15–16, Washington DC

Leete E 1988b The treatment of schizophrenia: a patient's perspective. Hospital and Community Psychiatry 38:486–491

Leete E 1989 How I perceive and manage my illness. Schizophrenia Bulletin 15:197–200

Leff J P, Vaughn C E 1985 Expressed emotion in families. Guildford Press, New York

Lefley H P 1989 Family burden and family stigma on major mental illness. American Psychologist 44:556–560

Lelliott P, Beevor A, Hogman G et al 1999 The CUES project. Carer and User Expectations of Services. A part of the Department of Health's SCA Initiative (Outcomes of Social Care for Adults). Final report. Royal College of Psychiatrists Research Unit/National Scizophrenia Fellowship, London

Lelliott P, Beevor A, Hogman G et al. 2001 Carers' and users' expectations of services – user version (CUES-U): a new instrument to measure the experience of users of mental health services. British Journal of Psychiatry 179:67–72

Lewis G, Sloggett A 1998 Suicide, deprivation and unemployment. Record linkage study. British Medical Journal 317:1283–1286

Lindow V 1994 Purchasing Mental Health Services: self-help alternatives. Mind Publications, London

Lindow V 1996 What we want from community psychiatric nurses. In: Read J, Reynolds J (eds) Speaking Our Minds. Open University Press, Milton Keynes, p 186–190

Lindsey H 1976 The Terminal Generation. Fleming-Revel, Old Tappan, NJ

Link B, Struening E L, Neese-Todd S et al 2001 The consequences of stigma for the self-esteem of people with mental illness. Psychiatric Services 52:1621–1626

Link B G, Phelan J C 2001 Conceptualising stigma. Annual Review of Sociology 27:363–385

Lovejoy M 1982 Expectations and the recovery process. Schizophrenia Bulletin 8:605–609

Luckstead A, Coursey R D 1995 Consumer perceptions of pressure and force in psychiatric treatments. Psychiatric Services 46:146–152

McCandless-Glincher L, McKnight S, Hamera E et al 1986 Use of symptoms by schizophrenics to monitor and regulate their illness. Hospital and Community Psychiatry 37:929–933

McDermott B 1990 Transforming depression. The Journal of the California Alliance of the Mentally Ill 1:13–14

McGlashen T H 1988 A selective review of North American long term follow up studies of schizophrenia. Schizophrenia Bulletin 14:515–542

McGrath M E 1984 First person accounts: where did I go? Schizophrenia Bulletin 10:638–640

McGuffin P, Owen M J, Farmer A E 1995 Genetic basis of schizophrenia. Lancet 346:678–682

McHarron A, Nettle M 1999 Guidance Paper 1: Payments to service users. West Midlands National Health Service Executive, Birmingham

Manic Depressive Fellowship 2001 Planning Ahead. Manic Depressive Fellowship, London

Manning C, White P D 1995 Attitudes of employers to the mentally ill. Psychiatric Bulletin 19:541–543

Marcel G 1962 Homo Viator (translated by E Crawford). Harper and Row, New York

May R 1999 My recovery journey. In: Proceedings of the Strangefish Conference: 'Recovery: An Alien concept' at Chamberlin Hotel, Birmingham, UK

May R 2000 Routes to recovery – the roots of a clinical psychologist. Clinical Psychology Forum 26:35–41

Meddings S, Perkins R 1999 Service user perspectives on the 'rehabilitation team' and roles of professionals within it. Journal of Mental Health 8:87–94

Menninger K 1959 Hope. American Journal of Psychiatry 116:481–491

Mental Health Foundation 2001 Is anybody there? A survey of friendship and mental health. Mental Health Foundation, London

Mental Health Task Force 1994 Building on experience: a training pack for mental health service users working as trainers, speakers and workshop facilitators. National Health Service Executive, London

Mental Health Task Force 1995 Black Mental Health – a dialogue for change. Department of Health, London

Miller J F 1985 Hope doesn't necessarily spring eternal – sometimes it has to be carefully mined and channelled. American Journal of Nursing January:23–24

Miller J F 1992 Coping With Chronic Illness: overcoming powerlessness, 2nd edn. Davis, Philadelphia

Mind 2001 Roads to Recovery. Mind Publications, London

Mirin S M, Namerow S M 1991 Why study treatment outcome? Hospital and Community Psychiatry 42:1007–1013

Morice R 1990 Cognitive inflexibility and pre-frontal dysfunction in schizophrenia and mania. British Journal of Psychiatry 157:50–54

Morice R, Delahunty A 1996 Frontal/executive impairment in schizophrenia. Schizophrenia Bulletin 22:125–137

Morris D 2001 Citizenship and community in mental health: a joint national programme for social inclusion and community partnership. The Mental Health Review 6:21–24

Moser K A, Goldblatt P O, Fox, ? ?, Jones D R 1987 Unemployment and mortality: comparisons of the 1971 and 1981 longitudinal study census samples. British Medical Journal 294:86–90

Mueller D 1980 Social networks: a promising direction for research on the relationship of the social environment to psychiatric disorder. Social Science and Medicine 14:147–161

Mueser K T, Bellack A, Blanchard J 1992 Comorbidity of schizophrenia and substance abuse: implications for treatment. Journal of Clinical and Consulting Psychology 60:845–855

Mueser K T, Bond G R, Drake R E, Resnick S G 1998 Models of community care for severe mental illness: a review of research on case management. Schizophrenia Bulletin 24:37–74

Murphy J M 1976 Psychiatric labelling in cross-cultural perspective. Science 191:1019–1028

National Alliance for the Mentally Ill 1996 Open Your Mind. Campaign pack, survey and insurance briefings. National Alliance for the Mentally Ill, Washington, DC

National Schizophrenia Fellowship 2000a Carer's Assessment Pack. National Schizophrenia Fellowship, London

National Schizophrenia Fellowship (in conjunction with Royal College of Psychiatrists Research Unit, Royal College of Nursing Research Institute and University of East Anglia Department of Social Work) 2000b CUES – service-user version. National Schizophrenia Fellowship, London

Nehring J, Hill R, Poole L 1993 Work, Empowerment and Community. Research and Development in Psychiatry (now The Sainsbury Centre for Mental Health), London

Nelson H 1997 Cognitive Behavioural Therapy with Schizophrenia. Nelson Thornes, London

Neuberg S L, Snith D M, Hoffman J C, Russell F J 1994 When we observe stigmatised and 'normal' individuals interacting: stigma by association. Personality and Social Psychology Bulletin 20:196–209

Nordt et al 2001 Recognition increases social distance: a dilemma for anti-stigma strategies. In: Proceedings of the World Psychiatric Association Conference, 'Together Against Stigma'. Leipzig, Germany

O'Donoghue D 1994 Breaking Down the Barriers. The stigma of mental illness: a user's point of view. The All Wales User Network, Aberystwyth, Wales

Office of National Statistics 2000 Labour Force Survey 1998/9. Office of National Statistics, London

O'Hagan M 1996 Two accounts of mental distress. In: Read J, Reynolds J (eds) Speaking Our Minds. Macmillan, London

Oliver M 1990 The Politics of Disablement. Macmillan, Basingstoke

Oliver N, Kuipers E 1996 Stress and its relationship with expressed emotion in community mental health workers. International Journal of Social Psychiatry 42:150–159

Onyett S, Heppleston T, Bushnell D 1994 A national survey of community mental health teams. Journal of Mental Health 3:175–194

Perkins R E 1992 Catherine is having a baby . . . Feminism and Psychology 2:56–57

Perkins R 1998 An act to follow? A Life in The Day 2:15–20

Perkins R E 1999 My three psychiatric careers. In: Barker P, Davidson B, Campbell P (eds) From the Ashes of Experience. Whurr Publications, London

Perkins R 2000 I have a vision … Open Mind 104:6

Perkins R 2001a All in a day's work. In: 'Just the Job' section. Evening Standard 8th October, p 15

Perkins R E 2001b What constitutes success? The relative priority of service users' and professionals' views of the effectiveness of interventions and services [editorial]. British Journal of Psychiatry 178:1–2

Perkins R 2001c Danger and incompetence: mental health and New Labour. Critical Social Policy 21:536–539

Perkins R E, Dilks, S 1992 Worlds apart: working with severely socially disabled people. Journal of Mental Health 1:3–17

Perkins R E, Goddard K 2002 Involving service users and their relatives. In: James A J B, Kendall T, Worrall A (eds) Clinical Governance in Mental Health and Learning Disability Services. Gaskell, London

Perkins R E, Repper J M 1996 Working Alongside People with Long Term Mental Health Problems. Stanley Thornes, Cheltenham

Perkins R E, Repper J M 1998 Dilemmas in Community Mental Health Practice. Choice or control. Radliffe Medical Press, Oxford

Perkins R, Repper J 2001 Exclusive language? In: Watkins C, Whitehead E (eds) Stigma and Social Exclusion in Healthcare. Routledge, London, p. 147–157

Perkins R, Evenson, E, Davidson, B 2000 The Pathfinder User Employment Programme. South West London and St. George's Mental Health NHS Trust, London

Perkins R, Evenson E, Lucas S, Harding E 2001a What sort of support in employment? A Life in the Day 5:6–13

Perkins R, Rinaldi M, Hardisty J 2001b User Employment Programme progress report 2001. South West London and St. George's Mental Health NHS Trust, London

Peters J 1997 Stigma and Discrimination Against People Who Have a Mental Illness: mental health organisation's views – a survey summary. Waitemata Health, Auckland

Pharoah F M, Mari J J, Steiner D 2001 Family intervention for schizophrenia (Cochrane Review). In: The Cochrane Library, issue 2. Update Software, Oxford

Philippe A 1988 Suicide and unemployment. Psychologie Medicale 20:380–382

Philo G, Henderson L, McLaughlin G 1993 Mass Media Representation of Mental Health/Illness: report for the Health Education Board for Scotland. Glasgow University, Glasgow

Picardie R 1998 Before I Say Goodbye. Penguin, Harmondsworth

Pilvin B 1982 And wisdom to know the difference. In: Shetler H, Straw P (eds) A New Day: voices from across the land. National Alliance for the Mentally Ill, Arlington, VA

Platt S, Kreitman N 1984 Trends in parasuicide among unemployed men in Edinburgh 1968–82. British Medical Journal 289:1029–1032

Plugge H 1979 Different hope. In: Fitzgerald R (ed) The Source of Hope. Pergamon, London

Podvoll E 1990 The Seduction of Madness: a compassionate approach to recovery at home. Century, London

Post F 1994 Creativity and Psychopathology: a study of 291 world-famous men. British Journal of Psychiatry 165:22–34

Post F 1996 Verbal creativity, depression and alcoholism: an investigation of one hundred American and British writers. British Journal of Psychiatry 168:545–555

Pozner A, Ng M, Hammond J, Shepherd G 1996 Working It Out: creating employment opportunities for people with mental health problems – a development handbook. Pavilion Publishing, Brighton

Pratt P 1998 The administration and monitoring of neuroleptic medication. In: Brooker C, Repper J (eds) Serious Mental Health Problems in the Community: policy, practice and research. Baillière Tindall, London

Read J, Baker S 1996 Not Just Sticks and Stones: a survey of the stigma, taboos and discrimination experienced by people with mental health problems. Mind Publications, London

Read J, Harre N 2001 The role of biological and genetic causal beliefs in the stigmatisation of 'mental patients'. Journal of Mental Health 10:223–235

Read J, Reynolds J 1996 Speaking Our Minds. Macmillan, London

Reeves A 1998 Recovery. A holistic approach. Handsell Publishing, Runcorn

Repper J 2000a Adjusting the focus of mental health nursing: incorporating service users' experiences of recovery. Journal of Mental Health 9:575–587

Repper J M 2000b Social Inclusion. In: Thompson T, Matthias P (eds) Mental Health and Disorder, 3rd edn. Baillière Tindall, London

Repper J, Cooke J, Ford R 1994 How can nurses build trusting relationships with people who have severe and long term mental health problems? Experiences of case managers and their clients. Journal of Advanced Nursing 19:1096–1104

Repper J, Sayce L, Strong S, Willmot J, Haines M 1997 Tall Stories from the Backyard. A survey of 'NIMBY' opposition to community mental health facilities experienced by key service providers in England and Wales. Mind Publications, London

Repper J, Perkins R, Owen S 1998 'I wanted to be a nurse...but I didn't get that far': women with serious ongoing mental health problems speak about their lives. Journal of Psychiatric and Mental Health Nursing 5:505–513

Repper J, Felton A, Hanson B et al 2001 One small step towards equality: involving service users in the education of mental health nurses. Mental Health Today December:7–9

Ridgeway P 1988 The Voice of Consumers in Mental Health Systems: a call for change. Center for Community Change through Housing and Support, Burlington, VT

Rinaldi M 2000 Insufficient Concern. Merton Mind, London

Rogers J 1995 Work is key to recovery. Psychosocial Rehabilitation Journal 18:5–10

Rogers A, Pilgrim D 1994 Service users' views of psychiatric nurses. British Journal of Nursing 3:16–18

Rogers A, Pilgrim D 1997 The contribution of lay knowledge to the understanding and promotion of mental health. Journal of Mental Health 157:539–550

Rogers E S, Chamberlin J, Ellison M L et al 1997 A consumer-constructed scale to measure empowerment among users of mental health services. Psychiatric Services 48:1042–1047

Rogers K 1957 The necessary and sufficient conditions of therapeutic personality change. Journal of Counselling Psychology 21:95–103

Romme M, Escher S 1993 Accepting Voices. Mind Publications, London

Romme M, Honig A, Noorthoorn E, Escher S 1992 Coping with hearing voices: an emancipatory approach. British Journal of Psychiatry 161:99–103

Rose D 1996 Living in the Community. Sainsbury Centre for Mental Health, London

Rose D 2001 Users' Voices. Sainsbury Centre for Mental Health, London

Rowland L A, Perkins R E 1988 You can't eat, drink or make love eight hours a day: the value of work in psychiatry. Health Trends 20:75–79

Ruggieri M 1994 Patients'and relatives' satisfaction with psychiatric services: the state of the art of its measurement. Royal College of Psychiatrists, London

Ruscher S M, de Wit R, Mazmanian D 1997 Psychiatric patients' attitudes about medication and factors affecting non-compliance. Psychiatric Services 48:82–85

Russinova Z 1999 Providers' hope-inspiring competence as a factor optimizing psychiatric rehabilitation outcomes. Journal of Rehabilitation 16:50–57

Ryan T, Bamber C 2002 Pricing Participation: a survey of organisational payment practices to users and carers for expenses and time given in service development and delivery. North West Mental Health Development Centre (part of the Institute for Applied Health and Social Policy, King's College, London), Manchester

Sackett D L 1976 The magnitude of compliance and non-compliance. In: Sackett D L, Haynes R B (eds) Compliance with Therapeutic Regimens. John Hopkins University Press Baltimore, MD, p 9–25

Sainsbury Centre for Mental Health 1997 Pulling Together: the future roles and training of mental health staff. Sainsbury Centre for Mental Health, London

Sandford T 1994 Users' perceptions of clinics providing depot phenothiazine treatments. In: Gournay K, Sandford T (eds) Perspectives on Mental Health Nursing. Scutari, London

Sartorius N 2000 Why bother about stigma because of schizophrenia? In: The Lily Psychiatry Lecture, Annual Meeting of the Royal College of Psychiatrists, Edinburgh, UK

Sartorius N 2001 Introductory remarks. In: Proceedings of the World Psychiatric Association Conference, 'Together Against Stigma', Leipzig, Germany

Sayce L 1997 Motherhood: the final taboo in community care. Women and Mental Health Forum 2:4–7

Sayce L 1998 Stigma, discrimination and social exclusion: what's in a word? Journal of Mental Health 7:331–343

Sayce L 2000 From Psychiatric Patient to Citizen. Overcoming discrimination and social exclusion. Macmillan, London

Sayce L 2001a Not just users of services, but contributors to society: the opportunities of the disability rights agenda. The Mental Health Review 6:25–28

Sayce L 2001b Psychiatric disability and the disability rights agenda. HAS Rehab Good Practice Network Newsletter 5:3–5

Sayce L 2002 Beyond Good Intentions: making anti-discrimination strategies work. Disability Rights Commission, London

Sayce L, Measey L 1999 Strategies to reduce social exclusion for people with mental health problems. Psychiatric Bulletin 23:65–67

Sayce L, Morris D 1999 Outsider Coming In: achieving social inclusion for people with mental health problems. Mind Publications, London

Scazufca M, Kuipers E 1999 Coping strategies in relatives of people with schizophrenia before and after psychiatric admission. British Journal of Psychiatry 174:154–158

Schmook A 1994 They said I would never get better. In: Spaniol L, Koehler M (eds) The Experience of Recovery. Center for Psychiatric Rehabilitation, Boston

Schradle S B, Dougher M J 1985 Social support as a mediator of stress: theoretical empirical issues. Clinical Psychology Review 5:641–646

Schulze B, Richter-Werling M 2001 'Crazy? So what!' Project weeks on mental health and illness. Their effects on secondary school students' attitudes towards people with schizophrenia. In: Proceedings of the World Psychiatric Association Conference, 'Together Against Stigma', Leipzig, Germany

Scott J, Seebohm P 2002a Payments and the Benefits System: a guide for survivors and service users involved in improving mental health services. Institute for Applied Health and Social Policy, King's College, London

Scott J, Seebohm P 2002b Payments and the Benefits System: a guide for managers paying service users involved in improving mental health services, London: Institute for Applied Health and Social Policy, King's College, London

Scott R R, Himadi W, Keane T M 1984 A review of generalisation in social skills training: suggestions for future research. Progress in Behaviour Modification 15:113–172

Secker J, Membury H 2000 'The Wicked Issues' in Wales. In: Proceedings of the Care Programme to Work Conference, Centre for Mental Health Services, Swansea, Wales. Centre for Mental Health Services Development, London

Secker J, Grove B, Seebohm P 2001 Challenging barriers to employment, training and education for mental health service users. The service users' perspective. Journal of Mental Health 10:395–404

Shepherd G 1977 Social skills training: the generalisation problem. Behaviour Therapy 8:100–109

Shepherd G 1978 Social skills training: the generalisation problem – some further data. Behaviour Research and Therapy 116:287–288

Shepherd G 1984 Institutional Care and Rehabilitation. Longman, London

Shepherd G 1989 The value of work in the 1980s. Psychiatric Bulletin 13:231–233

Shepherd G, Murray A, Muijen M 1995 Perspectives on schizophrenia: a survey of user, family care and professional views regarding effective care. Journal of Mental Health 4:403–422

Sherman P S, Porter R 1991 Mental health consumers as case management aids. Hospital and Community Psychiatry 42:494–498

Showalter E 1985 The Female Malady: women, madness and English culture 1830–1980. Virago, London

Simmons S 1994 Social networks: their relevance to mental health nursing. Journal of Advanced Nursing 19:283–289

Smith J, Birchwood M, Cochrane R, George S 1993 The needs of high and low expressed emotion families: a normative approach. Social Psychiatry and Psychiatric Epidemiology 28:11–16

Smith R 1985 'Bitterness, shame, emptiness, waste'. An introduction to unemployment and health. British Medical Journal 291:1024–1028

Social Exclusion Unit 1999 What's it all about? Available online: http://www.cabinet-office.gov.uk/seu/index/faqs.hmtl

Spaniol L, Koehler M 1994 (eds) The Experience of Recovery. Center for Psychiatric Rehabilitation, Boston

Spaniol L, Zipple A 1994 Coping strategies for families of people who have a mental illness. In: Lefley H, Wasow M (eds) Helping Families Cope With Mental Illness. Guilford Press, New York, p 178–190

Spaniol L, Gagne C, Koehler M 1997 Recovery from serious mental illness: what it is and how to assist people in their recovery. Continuum 4(4):3–15

Srebnick D, Robinson M, Tanzman B H 1990 Participation of mental health consumers in research: empowerment in practice. In: Proceedings of the Applied Psychology Association Convention, Boston, MA, USA

Steward 1996 Unemployment and health. 1. The impact on clients in rehabilitation and therapy. British Journal of Therapy and Rehabilitation 3:360

Stotland E 1969 The Psychology of Hope. Jossey-Bass, San Francisco

Strauss J S 1985 Negative symptoms: future developments of the concept. Schizophrenia Bulletin 11:3

Strauss J S 1994 The person with schizophrenia as a person II. Approaches to the subjective and complex British Journal of Psychiatry 164 (suppl 23):103–107

Szasz T 1961 The Myth of Mental Illness. Harper and Row, New York

Szmuckler G 1996 From burden to care giving. Psychiatric Bulletin 20:449–451

Tarrier N 1992 Management and modification of residual psychotic symptoms. In: Birchwood M, Tarrier N (eds) Innovations in the Psychological Management of Schizophrenia. John Wiley, Chichester, p 147–170

Tarrier N, Barrowclough C, Vaughn C 1988 The community management of schizophrenia: a controlled trial of behavioural interventions with families to reduce relapse. British Journal of Psychiatry 153:532–542

Taylor P, Gunn J 1999 Homicides by people with mental health problems: myth and reality. British Journal of Psychiatry 174:9–14

Thomas P 1997 The Dialectics of Schizophrenia. Free Association Books, London

Torrey E F 1983 Surviving Schizophrenia: a family perspective. Harper and Row, New York

Turner-Crowson J, Wallcraft J 2002 The recovery vision for mental health services and research: a British perspective. Psychiatric Rehabilitation 25:245–254

Unger K V, Anthony W A, Sciarappa M P H, Rogers S E 1991 A supported education programme for young adults with long-term mental illness. Hospital and Community Psychiatry 42:838–842

Unziker R 1989 On my own: a personal journey through madness and re-emergence. Psychosocial Rehabilitation Journal 13:71–77

Vaughn C, Leff J 1976a The measurement of expressed emotion in the families of schizophrenic patients. British Journal of Social and Clinical Psychology 15:57–65

Vaughn C, Leff J 1976b The influence of family and social factors on the course of psychiatric illness. British Journal of Psychiatry 129:125–137

Vincent S S 1999 Using findings from qualitative research to teach mental health professionals about the experience of recovery from psychiatric disability. In: Proceedings of the Harvard University Graduate School of Education Fourth Annual Student Research Conference, Cambridge, MA, USA, p 72–81

Voice Your Views 2000 Meetings Guidelines for Involving Mental Health Service Users in your Meetings. Service Users Reference Group, Avon and Western Wiltshire Mental Health National Health Service Trust, Bristol

Wallcraft J 2002 In my opinion we should abolish the Mental Health Act [opinion article]. Available online: http://www.scmh.org.uk/wbm23.ns4/WebLaunch/LaunchMe

Warner R 1985 Recovery From Schizophrenia. Psychiatry and political economy, 1st edn. Routledge, London

Warner R 1994 Recovery From Schizophrenia. Psychiatry and political economy, 2nd edn. Routledge, London

Warner R 2000 The Environment of Schizophrenia, Innovations in Practice, Policy and Communications. Routledge, London

Warr P 1987 Unemployment and Mental Health. Oxford University Press, Oxford

Wasow M 2001 Strengths versus deficits, or musician versus schizophrenic. Psychiatric Services 52:1306–1307

Watkins J 1996 Living With Schizophrenia. An holistic approach to understanding, preventing and recovering from negative symptoms. Hill of Content, Melbourne

Weiner S 1987 Bravado and the mental health clients' self-help movement. Hang Tough: Newsletter of the Marin Network of Mental Health Clients 2:6

Wertheimer A 1997 Images of Possibility: creating learning opportunities for adults with mental health difficulties. National Institute for Adult Continuing Education, Leicester

Williams A 1985 The value of QALYS. Health and Social Service Journal 94:3–5

Willick M 1992 Schizophrenia. A parent's perspective – mourning without end. In: Andreason N (ed) Schizophrenia From Mind to Molecule. American Psychiatric Press, London

Wilson Besio S 1987 The role of ex-patients and consumers in human resource development for the 1990s. Center for Community Change Through Housing and Support, Burlington, VT

Wilson S, Walker G 1993 Unemployment and health. A review. Public Health 107:153–162

Winefield H, Burnett P 1996 Barriers to an alliance between family and professional caregivers in chronic schizophrenia. Journal of Mental Health 5:223–232

Wing J K, Brown G W 1970 Institutionalism and Schizophrenia. Cambridge University Press, London

Wing J K, Morris B 1981 Handbook of Psychiatric Rehabilitation. Oxford University Press, Oxford

Woodside H, Landeen J, Kirkpatrick H et al 1994 Hope and Schizophrenia: exploring attitudes of clinicians. Psychosocial Rehabilitation Journal 8:140–144

World Health Organisation 1973 Report of the International Pilot Study of Schizophrenia. World Health Organisation, Geneva

World Health Organisation 1979 Schizophrenia: an international follow-up study. John Wiley, Chichester

Young S L, Ensing D S 1999 Exploring recovery from the perspective of people with psychiatric disabilities. Psychiatric Rehabilitation Journal 22:219–231

Zeitz M A 1995 The mothers' project: a clinical case management system. Psychiatric Rehabilitation Journal 19:55–62

Zubin J, Spring B 1977 Vulnerability – a new view of schizophrenia. Journal of Abnormal Psychology 86:103–126

Index

Index compiled by Lewis Derrick